Gourich

Forever Fit

A Step-By-Step Guide
for Older Adults

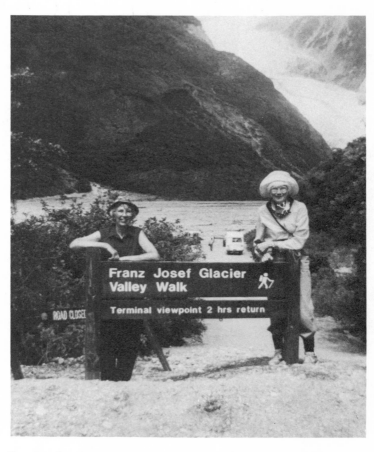

Staying fit, touring retirees enjoy a scenic New Zealand hike.

Forever Fit
A Step-By-Step Guide for Older Adults

Dee Ann Green Birkel, M.A.

Ball State University
Muncie, Indiana

and

Susan Birkel Freitag, M.S.

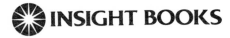 **INSIGHT BOOKS**

Plenum Press • New York and London

Library of Congress Cataloging in Publication Data

Birkel, Dee Ann Green.
    Forever fit: a step-by-step guide for older adults / Dee Ann Green Birkel and
Susan Birkel Freitag.
        p.   cm.
    "Insight books."
    Includes bibliographical references and index.
    ISBN 0-306-43969-7
    1. Physical fitness for the aged. I. Freitag, Susan Birkel. II. Title.
    [DNLM: 1. Exercise—in old age. 2. Health Promotion. 3. Physical Fitness. WE
103 B619f]
RA777.6.B56   1991
613.7'1'0846—dc20
DNLM/DLC   91-20810
for Library of Congress   CIP

The publisher and authors disclaim responsibility for any adverse effects or
consequences from the misapplication or injudicious use of the information
contained within this text.

ISBN 0-306-43969-7

© 1991 Plenum Press, New York
A Division of Plenum Publishing Corporation
233 Spring Street, New York, N.Y. 10013

An Insight Book

Printed in the United States of America

This book is dedicated to
our parents and grandparents,
whose lives were an example for us.

Preface

America is growing older. There are 24 million people over the age of 65 living in this country today. Furthermore, U.S. Census Bureau projections indicate that these numbers will increase dramatically in the next 50 years. Right now, there are more than 4 million people over age 80, and this number is expected to double by the year 2000. Not only is the general population growing older, but the older population is itself becoming older.

Contrary to popular belief, however, most older people are neither infirm nor institutionalized. In fact, only 5% of older Americans are living in institutions today, and of the 95% who are not, the majority (78%) declare their health to be "good" or "excellent." If you are in this group, this book is for you.

America is also growing more fit. It is estimated that 20% of Americans exercise regularly. And, just as Americans in general have become more conscious of the need to "stay fit," so too has this group of older Americans. Mature people have become increasingly aware of the benefits of physical fitness and increasingly interested in retaining their health, vitality, and physical attractiveness far into what used to be considered old age.

Sometimes, however, the need to do something becomes apparent long before the onset of old age. Even those who have generally been fit but are not currently exercising may, in their mid-40s or -50s, become aware of a shortness of breath that was not there 5 years ago, a constant dull ache in the shoulders or neck, a sharp twinge in the lower back, or a mounting feeling of fatigue. Then they may also feel the need to do something about the status of their physical well-being. If all this sounds familiar, this book is for you too.

Unfortunately, many people who are middle aged or older have had no formal training in exercise because it may not have been part of their school's curriculum. Although the desire to improve may exist, often the know-how does not. This book presents a nonthreatening but effective program of exercise for those who recognize the need to improve their physical well-being but who find many of the available classes, videos, and books on exercise unappealing. Although active aerobics classes in which already-fit young women perform vigorous dance routines may be fascinating to watch, they can, at the same time, be intimidating to those whose stamina and muscle tone are not what they once were and who may in fact approach the idea of a regular exercise program with hesitancy and a lack of confidence.

Unlike these programs, the exercise suggestions set forth in this book recognize that not all bodies are equal, that the body of an older person is not like that of a 22-year-old, and that a program of fitness for older persons requires a very special approach, tailored to the needs and interests of the more mature exerciser.

The purpose of this book is to provide a practical, step-by-step guide to health and physical fitness for older individuals who want to improve their physical potential. It evolved from our common professional backgrounds and interests, from our mutual interest in the health and well-being of our older parents, relatives, and friends, and from the awareness that we, too, are now on the brink of becoming older Americans.

Fortunately, there has never been a better time to be growing older. The youth-oriented society of the past 20 years is fading, and the intellectual, social, and physical options life offers for those over 50 are increasing. Suddenly, maturity is in. With this book we hope to help you explore the physical possibilities that life holds and to become the best you can be, whatever your age.

We begin by discussing the older population in general, the physical and social benefits of fitness to older adults, various dos and don'ts to consider before beginning, and how to set personal fitness goals. Next, we talk about the adaptations that can be made for those who, because of various physical limitations, are unable to follow a traditional program of exercise. We also look at the specific problems that sometimes accompany aging, such as osteoporosis, arthritis, and incontinence, and the effect many medications commonly used by older people have on exercise.

After a discussion of lifestyle and its effects on aging as well as a look at some basic guidelines, precautions, and techniques, we get into the exercises themselves. The section on building a stronger, more flexible body will serve as a basic reference for anything you choose to do. It presents clear, easy-to-follow directions for doing the exercises, along with detailed illustrations of each exercise. The book also includes a section on gentle muscle toning and strengthening exercises to be done in the water as well as a chapter on the "soft and gentle" exercises such as yoga and Tai Ji Chuan. Cycling, walking, dancing, and resistance exercises are all presented in separate discussions.

An important feature of the book is the format, which makes it easy to chart your progress and record health and exercise information. Included are a medical–exercise assessment form to be filled out by you and by your personal physician, temperature and humidity guides, and forms to be used for keeping a record of progressive conditioning. In addition, at the end of most chapters is a list of available resources and supplemental readings to help you maintain your new-found fitness and gain control over your life.

This book does not promise you the vigor and agility of someone 35 years your junior, but it will help you achieve your physical best as a mature, active person, and to enjoy yourself while doing it.

This is a good time to be growing older. But it is up to each one of us to make the process as personally productive, healthful, and exciting as we can. This book can help you reach these goals.

Acknowledgments

We wish to thank our family and friends who lent support and encouragement to us in writing this book.

Also a special thanks to our artist, Lydia Gerbig, for all the drawings; to Becky Birkel, R.Ac., for the section on acupuncture/ acupressure; to Tammy Hahn Birkel, R. Ph., and William Morton, M.D., for consultation about medications and exercise; to the participants in the Ball State University Retirees Exercise Program; and to our friends Gloriann Kalil and Janie Lewis, who read the early manuscript and encouraged us to pursue our dream of publication.

Contents

CHAPTER 1

Growing Old? So What!

> Growing old is inevitable for all of us. The clever
> thing is to accept it and always plan your next
> move well in advance.
>
> Maurice Chevalier

Growing old is becoming the rule rather than the exception in this country, but fortunately a great many people are actively and thoughtfully planning their "next move," into the third, or older, age. Happily, along with the increasing years have also come increasing opportunities and activities for older people, together with a greater interest in life and living, not just longer, but better.

The process of aging is ongoing and begins the moment we are born. From that moment, we are continuously growing older. For even in those that are healthy there is a steady physiological decline that begins at about 30 years of age and continues until the age of 80 or so. It is now widely believed, however, that inactivity, and not just age, contributes to this decline. How quickly the aging process takes place and how long it takes are not predeter-

mined. While genes do play an important part, we now know that
we have some control over the process of our own aging. We can
slow the whole thing significantly by looking at our lifestyle
carefully and making changes where necessary. Exercise is widely
believed to be one of the important ways we can change our life for
the better. Encouraging studies have shown that no matter when
in life a person begins to exercise, improvement can occur. It is
possible, even after years of inactivity, to join the ranks of the
"physically fit," a term that until only recently was applied almost
exclusively to the young. But fitness, like many other things, is
relative.

To say that someone is physically fit refers mainly to the
condition of his or her physical body, with respect to its flexibility,
muscular strength and endurance, agility, balance, and cardiorespiratory or aerobic capacity. The definition of fitness for older
adults is somewhat different, but in no way less accurate or
important. We describe fitness in midlife and beyond as the ability
to perform daily activities, maintain a healthful energy level, and
in general lead a life that brings enjoyment and satisfaction: one
that meets a person's physical, social, emotional, and intellectual
needs. What more can a person, at any age, ask of life?

EXERCISE AND YOU

Becoming physically fit, whether young or old, is not easy.
But it is not unbearably hard either. And there can be many
rewards: flexibility, weight loss, relief of pain or soreness, better
sleep, social interaction, and a more positive self-image. Imagine
your body right now at its personal best. Not the body of a 25-year-
old, but your own body, as a vigorous, vital, healthy, and attractive
person in his or her 50s, 60s, 70s, 80s, or even beyond. Visualize a
body that is more flexible, less overweight or fatigued, and per-

haps freer of pain or soreness. It is possible to have that body. Again, not a body that is unrealistically young, but one that best suits your age and physical capabilities. In spite of genes or chronological age, we can be better than we are right now, and exercise is one of the pathways to this goal.

PHYSICAL BENEFITS

Regular exercise can do a lot to help us reach our physical best and deal with the effects of growing older. For even though we may enjoy generally good health, it is only natural that as we grow older, each of us begins to experience, to varying degrees, some of the effects of aging. It may be a shortness of breath that wasn't there before, or an inability to do daily physical tasks with as much ease as was once possible. Or it may be an increasing blood pressure figure or a mounting feeling of fatigue. Finally, as we age, many of us experience pain. Not unbearable pain, but real pain, nevertheless, that makes it more and more difficult to hold onto a positive mental outlook. Often, this pain is the result of diminished flexibility or range of motion in our joints. Sometimes it results from muscles that have become so weakened that they cannot perform their usual function without painful consequences. Sometimes overweight is a factor, putting added strain and pressure on bones, joints, and muscles that are already weakened and performing less well than they should. And sometimes it is simply the result of disuse and lack of exercise.

This is unfortunate, because the good news is that many of the declines associated with aging can be put off or even prevented by regular exercise. So if a check with your physician indicates that there is no organic cause for your symptoms, perhaps an exercise routine that improves range of motion and flexibility will help you ease back into a more comfortable way of life: a way of life that allows you to maintain your independence and lessens the chance of home accidents, such as falls and burns, which often occur when an older person is in a weakened condition.

Almost any form of physical activity can help you overcome stress, increase your energy, and improve your health. A regularly scheduled workout, such as any of the programs we will describe in this book, is an excellent way to shape up. Many people who have begun such a program of exercise report the following benefits, among others: (1) increased muscle strength; (2) increased flexibility; (3) decreased blood pressure; (4) weight loss; and (5) improved circulation.

They also say that when they exercise, they often sleep better and have more energy to do their daily activities. Remember that exercise opportunities are there all the time, not only during your regularly scheduled work-out. Other unscheduled, spontaneous activities are also helpful. You are exercising whenever you mow the grass, work in the garden, do household chores, play a game of tennis or racquet ball, or walk up stairs instead of riding the elevator. All of these pleasant, day-to-day tasks and pursuits are "exercise" and play a part in your fitness routine.

As a final word of encouragement, some studies have shown (deVries, 1970) that a 70-year-old who exercises compares favorably physiologically to a sedentary 30-year-old. That should be incentive enough to get us up out of our chairs and into a more active way of life.

PSYCHOLOGICAL AND SOCIAL BENEFITS

Most people readily agree that exercise can improve our physical well-being at any age. We all know that while it is not the fountain of youth, it can definitely help a person to reach his or her own best physical state, regardless of age or disability. But the psychological and social benefits can be just as encouraging. Exercise can have a soothing yet energizing effect on our minds and spirits as well. It may possibly lengthen our lives, and it will certainly add to their quality.

Physical activity has been identified by Erdman Palmore as one of the predictors of "successful aging." In a study begun in 1955 at Duke University and continued for 21 years, successful aging was defined as survival to age 75 with good health and happiness. The 155 persons taking part in the study stated that the strongest factors contributing to their satisfaction with life were: (1) involvement in group activities and (2) physical activity.

Unfortunately, a much greater number of people are neither involved in groups nor taking part in physical activities, and so miss out on the satisfaction that accompanies them. Older people frequently cite lack of physical strength and energy as the main reason for not participating in pastimes they enjoy, but the very lifestyle they adopt, if it is one of passivity and inactivity, can be the culprit. Studies of healthy young men confined to bed or chair rest for as little as 3 weeks showed dramatic and distressing results: diminished ability to work, dizziness, nausea, vomiting, and circulatory collapse (Smith and Surfass, 1981). If this is true for healthy, young individuals, what must be the effect on the elderly? They may fall into a cycle of inactivity–fatigue–inactivity from which escape can be extremely difficult.

But escape is possible, as is, more importantly, prevention. The secret is regular physical activity and staying in the mainstream of life. In fact, Smith and Surfass state that exercise and the increase in energy that is often the happy result frequently allow older persons "to expand their daily activities out of the ordinary world of self care and basic sustenance into a more enriching atmosphere of more satisfying leisure pursuits " (pg. 124). There follows a trend away from an inactive, more sedentary way of life toward a more activity-oriented one, and this often results in new interests, new friends, and a greater joy in living.

MOTIVATION

Staying with an exercise program can be hard. Regular exercise, for all the good things it brings, can be difficult to fit into a busy schedule, expensive, boring, and physically taxing. So do not waste your time feeling guilty over lapses in your good intentions. You are not alone. The important thing is to get up out of your chair and begin again. Of course, you should check with your physician before you begin any program. Then, after you do, remember a few important points about sticking with an exercise program.

1. Choose something you like to do. No one is directing you to a specific activity. You are free to choose what you like. When you pick an activity that fits your lifestyle, interests, health and fitness needs, and personality, you are much more likely to stay with it.
2. Don't get carried away with your initial enthusiasm. Even though you may be highly motivated and eager to go, remember to start off slowly so that your body has time to adjust to its new physical regimen. Too much exercise at first will almost certainly dampen your enthusiasm, and may result in injury.
3. Be realistic about what you want to achieve, especially when it comes to weight loss and muscle toning. Allow at least a month of stretching and muscle-toning exercise before you look for significant improvements.

4. Exercise regularly. Intermittent spurts of activity do very little good. Plan on eventually doing 15–40 min three or four times a week.

5. Make time for exercise. Try to put a regular exercise period into your weekly schedule. If you have planned for exercise ahead of time, you will be less likely to find reasons for not doing it. But don't worry if you miss a day or two. Just begin again and get back on schedule. If time becomes a real problem, cut down on your routine rather than cutting it out altogether.

6. Try exercising with a partner. Working out with a spouse or friend can make the time fly and relieve the monotony. You will also be there to encourage each other when one of you feels like skipping a session.

7. Most of all, HAVE A GOOD TIME! It's hard to stay with anything that becomes a chore, and that is especially true of exercise. If you go into your exercise program keeping in mind all these pointers, it will be fun, and you will stick with it.

MAKE EACH DAY COUNT

There is no reason why the last years of our life should have any less meaning and potential for improvement and satisfaction than the first. There is no reason why we should look at our declining years as merely marking time. One thing is sure, whatever our age: Unless something unfortunate, such as serious illness or an accident, happens to us along the way, we are all journeying in the same direction: and that is toward being old. But it need not be a frightening trip. In fact, it is a stage in life where, with luck, we will all find ourselves eventually. Life is precious at any age, but it is our own responsibility to make it fulfilling and the very best it can be. Exercise is one way of doing this. So let's get started!

BIBLIOGRAPHY

References

deVries, H. A., and Hales, D., 1974, *Fitness After 50*, New York, Charles Scribner and Sons.

Palmore, E. B., 1979, Predictors of successful aging, *Gerontologist*, **19**(5):427–431.

Smith, E. L., and Surfass, R. C., eds., 1981, *Exercise and Aging: The Scientific Basis*, Hillside, N. J., Enslow Publishers.

Suggested Reading

Berger, S. M., 1989, *Forever Young*, New York, William Morrow and Company, Inc.

Brenton, M., 1989, *Aging Slowly*, Emmaus, Pa., Rodale Press.

Bricklen, M., 1990, How to buy a few extra years, *Prevention* **42**:144.

Brody, J. E., 1986, Aging: Studies point toward ways to slow it, *The New York Times*, Science Times, June 10, pp. 15, 18.

Clarkson-Smith, L., 1990, Aging smarter with exercise, *Prevention* **42**:12.

Drinkwater, B. L., 1988, Exercise and aging: The female masters athlete, in: J. L. Puhhl, et al., eds., *Sports Science Conference, November 30 to December 2, 1985*, Champaign, Ill., Human Kinetics Publishers, pp. 161–169.

Egginton, M., Kunigonis, M., Mintz, J., and Roser, D., 1984, *An Older Woman's Health Guide*, New York, McGraw-Hill Book Company.

Eichner, E. R., 1988, A profile of the mature athlete, in: W. A. Grana *et al.*, eds., *Advances in Sports Medicine and Fitness*, Chicago, Year Book Medical Publishers, pp. 1–21.

Fonda, J., and McCarthy, M., 1984, *Women Coming of Age*, New York, Simon and Schuster.

Freese, A. S., 1978, *The End of Senility*, New York, Arbor House.

Fries, J. F., 1989, *Aging Well*, Reading, Mass., Addison-Wesley Publishing Company.

Getchell, B., and Anderson, W., 1982, *Being Fit: A Personal Guide*, New York, John Wiley & Sons, Inc.

Hager, T., and Kessler, L., 1987, *Staying Young: The Whole Truth about Aging and What You Can Do to Slow Its Progress*, New York, Facts on File Publications.

Kapp, M. B., 1990, Empowering the elderly: dignity and health, *Current* **319**:10–13.

Kavanagh, T., and Shephard, R. J., 1990, Can regular sports participation slow the aging process? Data on masters athletes, *Physician and Sportsmedicine*, **18**:94–98; 101–102; 104.

Ley, O., 1984, *Exercises for Non-Athletes over Fifty-One*, New York, Random House.

Maxwell, R. B., 1990, AARP 90's goal—good health for all, *Modern Maturity* **33**:10–11.

Poppy, J., 1989, Thirty years of fortitude, *Esquire* **112**:83–85.

Rodale, R., 1990, Radical regeneration, *Prevention* **53**:30.

Rubenstein, C., 1990, Here's to your health, *New Choices for the Best Years* **30**:35–39.

Sneed, S. and Sneed, D., 1989, *Prime Time. A Complete Health Guide for Women 35–65*, Dallas, Word Publishing.

Winett, R. A., 1988, *Ageless Athletes: The Scientific Approach to Achieving High-Level Fitness and Counteracting the Effects of Aging*, Chicago, Contemporary Books.

Zuti, W. B., ed., 1984, *The Official YMCA Fitness Program*, New York, Rawson Associates.

CHAPTER 2

Getting Started
What You Need to Know

You cannot reach a goal unless you set one.
Unknown

Now that you have made the decision to alter your lifestyle by beginning an exercise program, you are ready to get started. This chapter and the ones to follow will provide the guidelines you need to safely start a program of appropriate exercise, and will offer suggestions for trying out a variety of suitable activities.

There are many reasons why a person may choose to exercise at home rather than as a part of a formal exercise class or group. Among these are: a lack of transportation, the cost of membership in a group, living in a remote area, a desire for privacy when exercising, or the need to be with an ill family member. Also, some people just feel more confident and less inhibited when they are not in a group setting. This book will help these people get into the exercise program they need without the necessity for a group. For those who would enjoy the social aspects of an exercise class but are prevented from attending one, a good alternative might be to invite a friend over to go through the exercises in this book together. Then, after a satisfying workout, a short visit and something to drink can provide the social benefits as well.

Whatever your reasons, if you are not to be part of a formal exercise group, this book will be a great help in answering your questions, planning your individual exercise program through questionnaires and checklists, keeping you motivated, and providing the means to record your activities and so chart your progress regularly. It will also serve as a good resource and reference book.

MEDICAL EVALUATION AND HEALTH HISTORY

The first step in any program of exercise is a thorough medical examination. Meet with your physician and discuss your intention to exercise, your present health status, and your health history. The AAHPERD Medical/Exercise Form (Fig. 2.1) will help you in this discussion. This form has been developed by physicians and professionals in the area of exercise and aging. The American Alliance of Health, Physical Education, Recreation, and Dance encourages its use by physicians to assist older adults in beginning an exercise program. The completed form should be used as a reference as you exercise at home. (Or, it could be given to the leader of an exercise class, should you plan sometime to join one.) See Appendix A for your personal copy to fill out and take to your physician.

AAHPERD Council on Aging and Adult Development
Medical/Exercise Assessment for Older Adults

Date _____

Name _____ Age _____ Phone (_____) _____
Street _____ City _____ State _____ Zip _____

Part 1—TO BE FILLED OUT BY PARTICIPANT

ACTIVITY HISTORY

1. How would you rate your physical activity level during the last year?
   _____ Little—Sitting, typing, driving, talking—no exercise planned
   _____ Mild—Standing, walking, bending, reaching, exercise 1 day per week
   _____ Moderate—Standing, walking, bending, reaching, exercise 1 day per week
   _____ Active—Light physical work, climbing stairs, exercise 2–3 days per week
   _____ Very active—Moderate physical work, regular exercise 4 or more days per week

2. What exercise and recreational activities are you presently involved in and how often? _____
   _____

HEALTH HISTORY

Weight _____ Height _____ Recent weight loss/gain _____
Please list any recent illnesses: _____
_____

Please list hospitalizations and reasons during last 5 years: _____
_____

Please check the box in front of those conditions which you have experienced.

☐ Anemia   ☐ Hernia
☐ Arthritis/bursitis   ☐ Indigestion
☐ Asthma   ☐ Joint pain in _____
☐ Blood pressure _____   ☐ Leg pain on walking
☐ Bowel/bladder problems   ☐ Lung disease
☐ Chest pains   ☐ Shortness of breath
☐ Chest discomfort while exercising   ☐ Passing out spells
☐ Diabetes   ☐ Osteoporosis _____
☐ Difficulty with hearing _____   ☐ Low back condition
☐ Difficulty with vision _____   ☐ Other orthopedic conditions [List]
☐ Dizziness or balance problems   _____
☐ Heart conditions _____

Figure 2.1. The AAHPERD Medical/Exercise Form. Developed by DeeAnn Birkel, Ray Harris, William Martz, and Wayne Osness.

Smoking:
  Never smoked   Smoke now [how much? _____]   Smoked in past
Alcohol consumption:
  None   Occasional   Often [how much? _____]
List any existing health concerns _____
_____

Please list medication and or dietary supplements you regularly take
_____

PART II—TO BE FILLED OUT BY PHYSICIAN
                                    Date of Last Examination _____

PHYSICAL EXAMINATION—Please check if it applies to the patient.

☐ Resting heart rate _____   ☐ Resting blood pressure _____
☐ Chest auscultation abnormal   ☐ Thyroid abnormal
☐ Heart size abnormal   ☐ Any joints abnormal
☐ Peripheral pulses normal   ☐ Abnormal mass
☐ Abnormal heart sounds, gallops   ☐ Other _____
Present prescribed medication[s] _____
_____

CARDIOVASCULAR LABORATORY EXAMINATION
[Within one year of the present date if recommended by physician].
DATE: _____

Resting ECG: Rate _____ Rhythm _____
  Axis _____ Interpretation _____
Stress test: Max H.R. _____ Max B.P. _____ Total time _____
  Max VO$_2$ _____ METS _____ Type of test _____
Recommendation for exercise. Moderate is defined as standing, walking, bending,
reaching and light exercise 3 days a week. Please check one.
_____ There is no contraindication to participation in moderate exercise program.
_____ Because of the above analysis, participation in a moderate exercise program
        may be advisable, but further examination or consultation is necessary,
        namely: stress test, EKG, other _____.
_____ Because of the above analysis, my patient may participate only under direct
        supervision of a physician. [Cardiac rehabilitation program]
_____ Because of the above analysis, participation in a moderate exercise program is
        inadvisable.

Figure 2.1. (continued)

SUMMARY IMPRESSION OF PHYSICIAN

Comments on any history of orthopedic and neuromuscular disorders that may affect participation in an exercise program—especially those checked. _____

_____

Message for the Exercise Program Director: _____

_____

Physician: _____ Signature: _____
      [Please type/print]

Address: _____ Phone: (_____) _____

PART III—PATIENT'S RELEASE AND CONSENT

_____ Release: I hereby release the above information to the Exercise Program Director.

_____ Consent: I agree to see my private physician for medical care and agree to have an evaluation by him/her once a year, if necessary.

SIGNATURE: _____ DATE: _____

Figure 2.1. (continued)

EXERCISE TERMINOLOGY

Some basic exercise terms need to be discussed now, before you go any further. Even if you are already familiar with these terms you should still read the following material because it contains information that pertains specifically to our bodies after age 45. This will help you to exercise the way you should now rather than as you did when you were 20— which may be inappropriate for the older you. Some of the terms you should be familiar with as you begin an exercise program follow.

Flexibility

Flexibility refers to the way a joint and the muscles that are attached to it move through a range of motion. Does the joint move freely or is it stiff? Stretching exercises that are static (which means thay are held and no bouncing is done) will help increase the length of a muscle or muscle group, thus improving flexibility.

Muscular Strength

Muscular strength is the muscle's ability to lift, move, or push against a resistant force. Sometimes the resistance is from the body itself and sometimes it is from an object such as a bicycle pedal or weight-resistance machine. The Overload Principle shows that a muscle can increase in size and strength when it is called upon to work at a greater-than-normal load. This is true for the muscle of the heart as well as for the muscles of the legs, arms, or any other part of the body.

Isometric

Isometric refers to the way a muscle contracts when working against a resistance that is fixed, and when the muscle does not change its length as it does in a stretching exercise. An example of this type of exercise would be when you hold your arms in front of your body with palms of the hands together and then push hard. The chest muscles, the pectorals, and the muscles of the arms contract but do not change length. This type of contraction increases the pressure in the chest and can elevate the blood pressure.

Isotonic

Isotonic also refers to the way the muscle contracts, but here the muscle changes length; it shortens. A good example of an isotonic exercise is when the arm is straight, you bend the elbow, and the biceps muscle then contracts and shortens. To work the muscle more you can hold an 8-oz can or a 1-lb weight. This added resistance will strengthen the muscle more.

Body Composition

Body composition refers to the proportion of body fat to lean body tissue, that is, your bones, muscles, internal organs: everything but fat. Being overweight is often associated with heart disease, high blood pressure, diabetes, gall bladder and kidney problems, and diseases of the joints. It can also cause complications in surgery. Further research needs to be done with older adults to develop recommendations as to what percentage of fat is considered normal for this older group. For younger people the acceptable range is 15% to 17% for men and 22% to 28% for women. Obesity is considered to be bodyfat over 30% for women and 20% for men. Our bodies change as we age and so does the distribution of fat on the body. Muscle weighs more than fat, so a person may gain weight when exercising because of an increase in lean body tissue, which is muscle, but may nevertheless lower the percentage of body fat. This is discussed further in the instructions for the Self-Appraisal Test, which appears later in this chapter. You can also ask your physician to measure your percentage of body fat.

Static Balance

Static balance refers to your ability to stand on one leg for a period of time without falling over. Roy L. Walford, in his book *The 120 Year Diet*, states that there is a 100% decline, from age 20 to age 80, in the ability to balance. Fortunately, balance is one area that is easily improved with practice. It is easy to incorporate some one-legged stands into your day. Practice standing on one leg while you are brushing your teeth, talking on the telephone, or standing at the kitchen sink. Doing the exercises for feet and legs, which are described in Chapter 6, will strengthen them and also help you improve your balancing ability.

Vital Capacity

Vital capacity refers to the amount of air the lungs bring in (inhale) and let out (exhale) during one breath. The amount declines as we age because of a lessening of elasticity in the lungs and the muscles of the rib cage. You will notice as you are learning the exercises that there is a prescribed breathing pattern. We urge you to follow this pattern because it will help you pace yourself and not go too fast during the exercise. It will also prevent your blood pressure from rising sharply. Being conscious of your breathing habits will encourage you to breathe deeply and help you maintain an adequate amount of air in your lungs and oxygen for your body.

Cardiorespiratory Efficiency

Cardiorespiratory efficiency refers to how well your lungs bring in the oxygen and how well your heart and vascular system transport this oxygen to your entire body. Cardiorespiratory efficiency can be determined in a laboratory or hospital by an exercise stress test on a treadmill or stationary bicycle. The amount of oxygen going into the body is known, and the amount being exhaled is measured; the remaining difference is what the body has kept to use and is called your "VO_2 Max." It is a good indicator of how physically fit a person is. This stress test, or exercise tolerance test as it is also called, measures the response of the heart and vascular systems under the stress of a heavy exercise load. This is done by means of electrodes attached to the body. The resultant electrocardiogram is then interpreted by the physician and the results made available to you. This test is recommended for everyone age 45 and older who is beginning an exercise program that will work the heart–lung–vascular system. The results of this test may be recorded on the AAHPERD Medical Assessment Form in this chapter (Fig. 2.1) and in Appendix A.

Warm up

The warm up is the beginning part of your exercise session and is composed of a series of exercises that prepares the body for its workout in a gentle manner that will stretch the muscles and increase the flow of blood to the joints and the muscles being used. It is most important to do this, because warming up can help prevent injury. When you begin to sweat and feel warm you are ready for the next part of your exercise routine.

Aerobic Workout

The aerobic workout refers to the main part of your exercise session. In this part you strive to exercise the heart muscle by doing an activity that is rhythmic and continuous; for example, walking, cycling, or swimming. This is explained further in the discussion of the physical fitness prescription factors that follows. Please remember that you should always be able to carry on a conversation or talk or sing to yourself during your exercise activity. Don't work so hard that your heart beats too rapidly or you become out of breath.

Cool down

The cool-down part is the continuation of some slower-paced activity done at the end of an exercise session to cool down the body gradually. This facilitates the flow of blood from the extremities and assists the cardiorespiratory system in returning to a lower pulse and respiratory rate. It also prevents the accumulation of lactic acid in the muscles, which is thought to be a contributing factor in muscle soreness.

PHYSICAL FITNESS PRESCRIPTION FACTORS

The following elements should be considered when deciding upon an exercise program either as part of a group or when setting up your own. Just as a physician prescribes medicines, so exercise can also be prescribed.

Intensity

The pulse rate is used to indicate how hard the exercise session should be. A beginner or sedentary person is safe with an exercise pulse rate of 20 beats above the resting pulse. Roy Shepherd, an exercise physiologist, recommends working at a level of 40% of the maximum pulse for a longer period of time.

Others recommend 50% to 60% of the maximum heart rate for those who have a more active lifestyle and who have no history of heart disease. The rate of perceived exertion is also a means of determining the intensity of a workout. This and the formula for determining the target heart rate will be discussed in Chapter 5.

Duration

The recommended amount of time spent in exercise for a beginner or sedentary person is 5 to 10 min a day, working up to 15 to 30 min of continuous daily activity. This gentle approach lets the body begin its adjustment to exercising without causing injury or overexertion. A person who has been exercising regularly (for instance, walking every day) would probably be comfortable and safe with walking longer than 15 to 40 min. Just remember, always do what feels comfortable for you.

Frequency

The recommended number of exercise days per week is two for the beginner or sedentary person, progressing to four within three to four weeks. It is beneficial to do some gentle stretching and strengthening exercises every day, however.

Type of Activity

The activity you choose should be of a continuous type. Walking, swimming, and water exercises are highly recommended, as are cycling, dancing, and yoga. Tai Ji Chuan, a controlled movement routine from China, is also becoming popular.

ESTABLISHING PERSONAL GOALS

As you think about what type of exercise program you will undertake, think first about what you would like to get out of it personally. It will be helpful, before you ever begin, to ask yourself the following questions (Table 2.1) about your attitudes toward exercise and your expectations from it.

TABLE 2.1
Personal Goals Record Form

Do I want to exercise with other people or do I prefer to exercise by myself?

What are my personal goals?

_____ I need to lose weight

_____ I hope to improve flexibility in my _____, _____, or _____

_____ I want to relieve pain in my _____, _____, and _____

_____ Other

I need to tone and strengthen the muscles in my

_____ abdomen	_____ feet
_____ thighs	_____ back
_____ arms	_____ neck and shoulders

Do I need to improve my balance? _____

Do I need to improve my agility and coordination? _____

Do I want a set of exercises I can do in privacy? _____

Do I need to learn to handle stress in my life? _____

I like to

_____ swim	_____ cycle
_____ walk	_____ do chair exercises
_____ dance	_____ do floor exercises
_____ play tennis	

What else do I want to gain from exercising? _____

_____

_____

BALL STATE UNIVERSITY SELF-APPRAISAL

Before you begin to exercise it is a good idea to have an overall picture or profile of your physiological status. The group of tests presented in this chapter and the form for recording the results (see Appendix B) will help you choose the physical activities that your body needs and from which you will gain the most benefit. By gathering this information at the beginning of your exercise regimen and once a month thereafter, you will be able to keep track of the progress you are making. Each test item will be discussed thoroughly, as will the correct techniques for performing the tests and gathering and recording your results.

Test 1: Resting Pulse

The pulse is an indication of how hard your heart and vascular system are working. A true resting pulse should be taken in the morning before you get out of bed. Locate your pulse either on the carotid artery in your neck or on the radial artery at the wrist (Fig. 2.2). Do not use the thumb to feel your pulse; only the index and

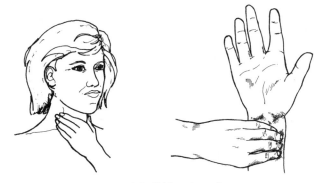

Figure 2.2. Taking the pulse.

middle fingers should be placed over the pulse area. Count for 30 sec, multiply this number by 2, and you will have your resting pulse rate for 1 min. Record this on your sheet.

Test 2: Height

Measure your height by standing erect against a wall in bare feet. Have someone mark where the top of your head is in line with the wall. One of the physiological changes of aging is that people (especially women) lose from 1 to 3 in, and possibly more, in height. This "shrinkage" takes place in the vertebral column or spine where the intervertebral discs are thinner as a result of compression or a reduction of fluid in the discs, making them less plump. When people begin to exercise, their overall muscle tone improves and thus their posture often improves as well. This is sometimes reflected in a slight increase in height.

Test 3: Weight

Weigh yourself in the morning before eating and dressing so that any changes in your weight will be accurate, and not the result of having just eaten or put on heavy clothes. Remember that muscle weighs more than fat, so a vigorous exercise program may yield a firmer, trimmer body without a significant weight loss.

Test 4: Blood Pressure

This is a measure of the blood flow as it is exerted against the artery wall. The systolic pressure, the high or top number, is the pressure measured at the moment the heart ejects blood (contracts). The diastolic pressure, the lower or bottom number, is the pressure measured when the heart is relaxed between beats. A reading of 140/90 or more is considered to be high blood pressure. Hypertension is the term used when the pressure starts high and stays high during rest. Research has shown a relationship between a systolic reading of more than 150 and a higher risk of heart attack than when the systolic pressure is under 120. Exercise helps to reduce the arterial pressure in some people. While it is normal for blood pressure to rise within a limited range during exercise, it should then lower following exercise.

It is important to monitor your blood pressure regularly. Many communities have free periodic checks, shopping malls often have machines to check your own blood pressure, and it is also possible to purchase instruments to check your blood pressure at home.

Test 5: Girth Measurements

If you are measuring yourself, keep the tape measure level and try to measure at the same body site each time. Pull the tape taut, and lap one end over the other to get an accurate reading. Make sure you are not measuring over bulky clothing or your finger. Always measure your right arm and leg. When taking your measurements, follow the positioning of the tape as illustrated in Figure 2.3.

Recommended girth measurements depend on an individual's body build. Again, most of the recommendations available are for the younger body and do not take into consideration the changes in the body as we go through life. But you can monitor the changes in your own body by taking your girth measurements periodically.

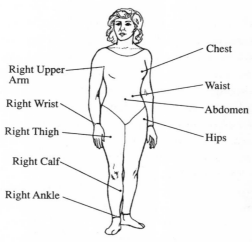

Figure 2.3. Girth measurements.

Test 6: Percentage of Body Fat

Finding out how much of the body is fat is considered the most accurate way to determine the body's healthy composition. Inexpensive instruments (see Resources) can be ordered to measure skinfold; or you can ask your physician to measure your body fat. Charts are available to convert the readings in millimeters shown on the calipers, or measuring instrument, to percentages. The old saying about "pinching an inch" (that is, 26 mm) indicates the upper limit of a safe percentage of fat. Unfortunately, most of the research on percentage of body fat has also been done on younger people, so there is a need for more work among the population over age of 58 years. Available studies have suggested that the percentage for men should be under 20% and that for women under 30%. However some researchers think this figure is too high.

Test 7: Flexibility of Back and Hamstrings

To check your flexibility in these areas you will need a chair, a footstool, or a bench laid on its side, as well as a yardstick or meterstick placed on the edge of the chair with the 10-in mark on the yardstick (or the 25.5-cm mark on the meter stick) lined up with the edge of the chair seat (Fig. 2.4). Please follow these instructions:

1. Do a few stretching exercises to gently warm up the muscle groups of the back and legs.
2. Remove shoes and wear loose clothing.
3. Sit on the floor, placing the soles of your feet against the chair seat and keeping your legs straight.
4. Place fingertips on your shoulders, inhale, and reach toward the ceiling, straightening arms, lifting ribs, and contracting the abdominal muscles. Then EXHALE and lean forward as far as you can comfortably reach WITH-OUT bending your knees. Read the number on the measuring stick where your fingertips touched. If it is above the 10-in mark, subtract 10 from the number and write down + _____. If you touched a number from 1 to 10, subtract your number from 10 and write down − _____.

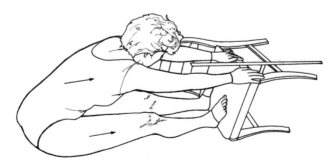

Figure 2.4. Flexibility.

Test 8: Balance

Wearing shoes with low heels, stand on one leg for 15 sec with other leg extended back (Fig. 2.5). As you test your ability to maintain your balance, try to do the following: Stand on one leg for 15 sec, showing control and steadiness and using arms and vision to balance effectively while in good form. Repeat this test every month or so, and record any improvement you notice.

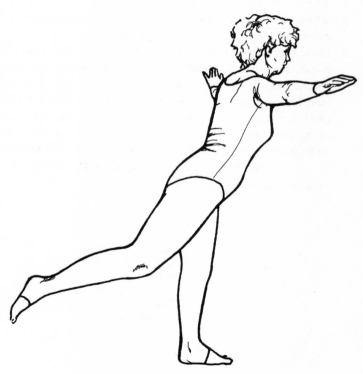

Figure 2.5. Balance.

Test 9: Cardiovascular Fitness

If you are able to walk either a half mile or one mile, you are encouraged to do one of these tests. Do the test you choose on a route that is measured accurately, or go to a school track, which is usually one fourth of a mile. Immediately upon completing either two laps (½ mile) or four laps (1 mile), take your pulse for 6 sec and add a zero. If you have walked a mile refer to the charts from the Rockport Walking Institute (Appendix C) to determine your aero-

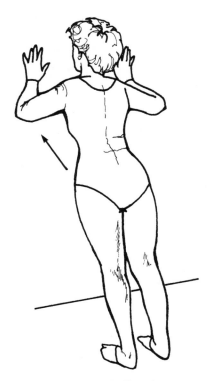

Figure 2.6. Wall push-up.

bic fitness level for your age group and sex. There are no norms available for the half-mile distance. As you continue to exercise you will see improvement and will increase your distance until you are walking one mile and can then do the Rockport Test.

Test 10: Arm Strength

This 15-sec wall push-up will test the strength in your arms. Stand facing a wall, about 3 feet away from the wall. Keep your feet flat on the floor and your body straight, with your hands, palms to the wall, slightly wider apart than your shoulders (Fig. 2.6). Count how many times you can bring your straight body forward to the wall in 15 sec. Keep breathing as you do this exercise; do not hold your breath. If you have arthritis in your arms or shoulders you may not want to do this test.

Test 11: Abdominal Strength Curl

Lie on your back, knees bent, with your fingertips on the floor touching a tape line. Note the number where you started. Curl

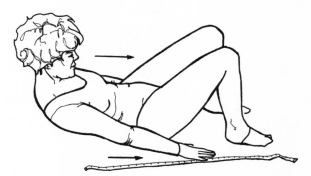

Figure 2.7. Abdominal strength curl.

and lift trunk, slide the fingers forward, and hold for a count of 5 (Fig. 2.7). Record the number of inches beyond your starting point that your fingers touched.

SUMMARY

Now that you have completed this self-appraisal you know more about your body's composition, your ability to balance and bend forward, and your muscular strength and aerobic capacity. Using the AAHPERD Medical/Exercise Form, you and your physician assessed your health and medical status. You also examined your own personal exercise goals. Since aging is often accompanied by medical conditions that may have an influence on your exercise plan and may prevent some of the more traditional exercises, this is a good time to look at some of these special problems and the exercise adaptations designed to assist you.

BIBLIOGRAPHY

References

Clark, B., 1986, Exercise Programs for Older Adults–What They Should Know to Get Started, *Journal of Physical Education, Recreation and Dance,* **57**(10):63–65.

Bouchard, C., and Despres, J. P., 1989, Variation in fat distribution with age and health implications, in: W. W. Spirduso and H. Eckert, eds., *Physical Activity and Aging: The Academy Papers of The American Academy of Physical Education,* Champaign, IL, Human Kinetics Publishers, Inc., pp. 78–106.

Eckert, H. M., 1989, Balance—To stand or fall, in: W. W. Spirduso and H. Eckert, eds., *Physical Activity and Aging: The Academy Papers of the American Academy of Physical Education,* Champaign, IL, Human Kinetics Publishers, Inc., pp. 37-41.

Lohman, T. G., Roche, A. F., and Martorell, R., eds., 1988, *Anthropometric Standard-ization Reference Manual*, Champaign, IL, Human Kinetics Publishers, Inc.

Osness, W., 1989, Assessment of physical function among older adults, in: D. K. Leslie, ed., *Mature Stuff: Physical Activity for the Older Adult*, Reston VA, American Alliance of Health, Physical Education, Recreation, and Dance/ Council on Aging and Adult Development, pp. 93–115.

Rippe, J. M., and Ward, A., 1989, *Rockport Walking Program*, New York, Prentice Hall Press.

Rossman, I., 1977, Anatomic and body composition changes with aging, in: Finch, C. E., and Hayflick, L., eds., *The Biology of Aging*, New York, Van Nostrand Reinhold, pp. 214–215.

Steen, M., 1988, Body composition and aging, *Nutrition Reviews*, **46**(2):45–51.

Van Camp, S. P., and Boyer, J. L., 1989, Exercise guidelines for the elderly, *The Physical and Sports Medicine*, **17**(5):83–86.

Suggested Reading

Harris, S. S., Caspersen, C. J., DeFriese, G. H., Estes, E. H., Jr., 1989, Physical Activity Counseling for Healthy Adults as a Primary Preventive Intervention in the Clinical Setting—Report for the US Preventive Services Task Force, *Journal of American Medical Association*, **261**:3590–3598.

Osness, W. H., 1986, Physical Assessment Procedures: The Use of Functional Profiles, *Journal of Physical Education, Recreation and Dance*, **57**(1):35–38.

Resources

Fat-O-Meter, plastic construction. Can be ordered from Sportime, One Sportime Way, Atlanta, GA 30340-1402.

CHAPTER 3

Special Conditions and Exercise Adaptations

Age . . . is a matter of feeling, not of years
George William Curtis

Even in today's activity-oriented society with its huge emphasis on fitness, health, and personal well-being, we must remember that for some individuals, a traditional exercise program is not recommended. Certain physical conditions contraindicate, or advise against, a general program of physical activity. Realistically, the many and varied health problems that sometimes accompany aging are a limiting factor for some. This does not mean, however, that a person must remain inactive, in pain, or out of shape. There are many ways of maintaining fitness and there are appropriate exercises for specific physical or medical conditions. Rather than not exercise, those with special health problems should especially be encouraged to participate safely in activities that are appropriate for their physical and medical status.

33

The elderly need special consideration and careful instruction from a trained professional who is knowledgeable about their health problems. Prevention of injury to the connective tissues is a major concern, as are health problems arising from heart and circulatory disorders. Keeping a positive outlook about exercise is always important: and especially so for older individuals or those with special health-related conditions.

A list of medical conditions that may limit your involvement in an exercise program of a traditional nature follows. A discussion of normal aging changes and medical conditions is presented and Table 3.1 suggests appropriate exercises for each condition. As always, it is recommended that you check with your doctor before you begin any exercise program, especially if you have any of these conditions.

Alzheimer's Disease

This is a disorder of the brain that causes loss of memory or serious mental deterioration. The nerve endings in the brain's outer layer, the cortex, degenerate and thus the passage of the electrochemical signals between the cells is disrupted. The diagnosis of this disease results after all other known causes of memory loss, such as hardening of the arteries, have been ruled out. There is no cure for the disease at present, but medical care can assist the person and the family in coping with the illness.

Maintaining physical activity is recommended, but if other health problems such as high blood pressure, osteoporosis, or heart disease exist, special considerations for those must be included in the exercise program as well. One advantage of a regular exercise session is that the caregiver can also benefit from the activity.

A list of some easy-to-follow suggestions and exercises for both patient and caregiver follows. The person with Alzheimer's Disease can imitate the activities; however, as the disease progresses they should be changed from 3- and 4-step sequences to 1-step repetitive activities. Refer to the Basic Warm-up Program (Chapter 6) for exercises and modify them as needed for the person with whom you are exercising.

1. Check with a medical doctor first about plans to exercise.
2. Set up a routine and repeat the exercise session at the same time of day, four or five days a week.
3. Play music that may be familiar and emotionally comforting, such as Sousa marches or Glen Miller songs. This can help create a happier environment.
4. Take long, brisk walks together for 30 min or more, four to five days a week. Encourage the patient to notice the environment, the birds singing, or the neighbors.
5. Practice deep breathing several times a day to increase the oxygen supply to the body.
6. Assist them by putting their arms, legs, and head into the position of the exercises; gently guide them in executing the activity if this is needed.
7. Continue the movement long enough so they can have a feeling of success.
8. Keep the verbal directions simple and repeat the same words. If there is no comprehension, try rephrasing the cues.
9. Smile and let the exercise time together be enjoyable. Whatever is accomplished is better than not doing anything at all.
10. Use props such as sponge balls, bean bags, balloons, or towels.
11. Continue the following activities as long as the person is able to do them: dancing, swimming, golf, biking, and even basketball and tennis.
12. Always stimulate the other senses when exercising: touch, through the use of props; hearing, using music; vision, doing eye–hand coordination exercises with bean

bags and balloons; and smell, burning incense during the
exercise session.
13. Be patient and tell yourself that you both are benefiting
from this exercise time together.

Many states have support groups with local chapters that
meet monthly. Many good books have been published to assist the
caregiver in caring for and coping with the person with Alzheimer's
Disease. Check the Resources Section for further information.

Arthritis

Exercise cannot cure arthritis, which is an inflammation of
the joints, but it can increase joint mobility and help you improve
your range of motion. If a joint is swollen and painful, do not try to
exercise that area, but try doing slow stretching exercises as soon
as you are able. This will gradually increase the strength and the
endurance of your muscles and the range of motion at the joint.
Definitely stay away from activities like jogging, weight lifting,
tennis, or racquetball, or anything else that involves sudden jerky
movements that put strain on joints. If you have rheumatoid
arthritis it would be best for you, your physician, and a physical
therapist to develop a personalized program for you. For more
information about arthritis refer to the Resources for the address
of the Arthritis Foundation.

Diabetes

This disease is characterized by an excessive discharge of
urine from the body. The incidence of diabetes is higher in the
older age groups and also among obese people. Patients with
diabetes must pay careful attention to medication, exercise, and
diet and remain on the alert for possible complications. Exercise

can stimulate the body to make better use of the insulin it produces and in this way helps counteract the effects of diabetes. It can also prevent excessive weight gain, which is sometimes a contributing factor in diabetes. In some persons who have experienced the onset of diabetes as adults, regular exercise may reduce or eliminate the need for medication. When exercising, it is wise to have a quick source of sugar readily available. If you are a diabetic it is most important that you discuss your exercise plans thoroughly with your physician.

Cardiovascular Diseases

Although cardiologists are not in complete agreement among themselves about the type and amount of exercise allowable for those with heart disease, moderate exercises such as swimming, walking, or water exercises have become more and more important in the rehabilitation and recovery plan of these patients. It is now strongly believed by most researchers that a program of regular, moderate exercise provides protection against further problems. Research has also shown that regular exercise can help reduce blood pressure—not during the exercise time itself, but overall. However, if you suffer from any type of cardiovascular disease, always check with your physician before beginning any program of exercise. Many communities have available the cardiac rehabilitation program, which is a medically supervised exercise program for those who have had heart attacks or are recovering from surgery.

Hernia

Hernias are tears in the tissue of the abdominal wall. A hiatal hernia occurs when the stomach protrudes into the chest cavity through a hole in the diaphragm. Many older people are afflicted with this condition. A program of gentle exercise tones the abdominal muscles and helps to prevent further progression of this condition.

Incontinence

This inability to maintain control over the bladder is frequently related to loss of support for the bladder. In women pregnancy often causes muscles, ligaments, and other tissues to stretch. When they fail to return to their previous state, stress incontinence is the result. The loss of urinary control can sometimes be linked directly to a weakened pubococcygeus (PC) muscle and the gradual weakening of the pelvic floor. Research has indicated that practicing PC exercises regularly may help prevent stress incontinence and may even alleviate symptoms. These exercises are known as Kegel exercises, so named for the University of Southern California gynecologist, Arnold Kegel, who developed them for patients who were to have surgery for a lack of bladder control.

Because loss of bladder control is an embarassing and uncomfortable condition (although not an uncommon one), it warrants further discussion plus a clear explanation of the exercises necessary to help regain control. To isolate the PC muscle, do the following test: While sitting on the toilet, stop and start the flow of urine three times. Then empty the bladder completely.

A description of the Kegel exercises follows. Now do the exercises, either sitting or lying down.

1. *Flicks*: Contract and release the PC muscle in time to your heartbeat.
2. *Holds*: Contract the PC muscle and hold for 10 sec. At the end, squeeze once more, harder and deeper, then release for 10 sec.

3. *Bear downs*: Bear down for 3 sec, relax, and repeat. (Note: If you are a woman with pelvic weaknesses, do not try these.)
4. *Gradual holds*: Slowly, over 10 sec contract the PC muscle to maximum, and then slowly reduce the tension in the muscle for 10 sec.

Research has also shown that doing the Kegel exercises has aided men in maintaining erections and increasing their control of orgasm. The practice of these exercises may also improve sexual function in women.

Obesity

This is generally considered to be an excessive amount of body fat. It is usually agreed that the most successful way to lose weight and keep it off is a combination of diet and exercise. Exercise can play an extremely important part because it results in the loss of body fat rather than lean muscle tissue. When you only diet, you lose both. So, even though your total weight decreases, so does your amount of important muscle tissue. With exercise in your weight-loss plan you not only preserve that muscle tissue, you also build it up. Exercise in the water (Chapter 12), when possible, is recommended for those who are overweight, as the water supports 85% of your body weight. Walking and riding an exercise bicycle (Chapters 9 and 10) are additional suggestions for those who are overweight or obese. Riding an exercise bicycle can be done in the privacy of your home.

Osteoporosis

This is a thinning condition of the bones, predominant in women, in which the bones become less dense and more porous.

One of the causes is thought to be inadequate calcium intake throughout a women's lifespan, and especially just before and following menopause. Everett Smith has conducted research with exercise participants at the University of Wisconsin and has discovered that each bone is strengthened by the movement of the muscles and ligaments that attach to that bone. It is now believed that weight-bearing exercises that increase muscle movement against the bone (walking, jogging, low-impact aerobics, arm and back exercises) can often prevent or slow this bone loss. Those with osteoporosis should avoid activities where there is a risk of falling, such as skating, road cycling, and walking where the surface is uneven and poorly lighted. They should also avoid doing any fast, jerky, or jarring movements.

Ulcers

Ulcers are irritations on the lining of the digestive tract and are worsened by stress, so, it is reasonable to assume that stress-reducing activities such as regular exercise and relaxation will lessen the problem and allow the body to heal more readily. Sometimes doing exercises lying on the floor will cause discomfort and maybe nausea.

Vision Problems

Two very common problems of aging are cataracts and glaucoma. Cataracts develop when the lens of the eye becomes cloudy and light rays are unable to pass through the lens to the retina. The modern surgical treatment, which evacuates the cloudy lens and implants a new one, is highly successful. Immediately following this surgery, there should be no sudden movements or exertion, and the head should not be lowered. Exercise is not recommended until the physician finds that the eye is completely healed. Glau-

Table 3.1
Suggested Activities for Specific Conditions

RECOMMENDATION: See your physician to discuss your choice of activity if you have any of the following conditions:

Condition	Try	Avoid
Arthritis	Slow, full-range-of-motion exercises Balance exercises Walking Posture exercises Swimming and water exercises in warm water Cycling Tai Ji Chuan Hatha yoga Chair exercises	Quick, jerky exercises Heavy weight lifting Jogging
Diabetes	Hatha yoga Walking Swimming Slow, continuous, rhythmic activities (have a quick source of sugar available)	Blisters on feet
Cardiovascular diseases Hypertension Atherosclerosis Arteriosclerosis Angina Congestive heart failure	Always do a 10–15 min warm up and cool down Swimming and water exercises Cycling Dancing Hiking with friend Hatha yoga	Having head lower than body for too long Prolonged arm exercises Heavy weight lifting or any other brief, intense physical exertion Heavy exertion in hot or cold weather or after a heavy meal

(continued)

Table 3.1. (Continued)

Condition	Try	Avoid
Cardiovascular diseases (continued)	Tai Ji Chuan Mall walking Always pace yourself Stop if you feel pain	
Heart attack	Cardiac rehabilitation program Walking Golf Swimming and water exercises Hatha yoga	Same as those listed for cardiovascular diseases
Hernia	Walking Hatha yoga Swimming and water exercises Gentle exercises to tone abdominals	Inverting the body; head lower than chest. Exercises that require strong abdominal contractions
Incontinence	Kegel exercises Moderate elevation of legs and pelvis Swimming and water exercises Walking	Jumping, weight lifting or any exercises that cause strain

Condition	Recommended Exercises	Exercises to Avoid
Obesity	Hatha yoga Tai Ji Chuan Exercise bicycle (larger seat) Swimming and water exercises Walking	Strenuous, weight-bearing exercises
Osteoporosis	Walking Modified wall push-ups Hatha yoga Tai Ji Chuan Exercise through the full range of motion at the joints	Jumping, quick jerky movements Anything with a risk of falling, e.g., skating
Ulcers	Walking Cycling Swimming Hatha yoga Tai Ji Chuan	Exercises that bring blood to the stomach
Vision problems Glaucoma Retina problems Eye surgery	Exercises to move eyes up, down, side-to-side, and in a circle Walking Tai Ji Chuan Exercise bicycle	Having head lower than body which increases pressure to the eyes

coma develops when there is an elevated fluid pressure within the eye, with resulting loss of vision and sometimes nausea and pain. Activities that increase the pressure to the eye, such as bending over for an extended period, should be avoided.

MEDICATIONS AND EXERCISE

When beginning an exercise program, it is very important for you to talk with your physician about any medications you are taking and how they will affect your exercise program. Since you may be taking medications of one kind or another, it is important that you be aware of any side effects that relate to exercise. Table 3.2 presents a detailed list of medication types (not brand names) that are the more commonly prescribed medications, then explains their effect on the body, and outlines precautions that should be taken when exercising. Please show this chart to your physician and discuss the medications you are taking so you will have a better understanding of the effect of your medications upon your exercising body.

SUMMARY.

Regular exercise not only keeps those who are well healthy and fit, it may also serve as a remedy for various medical conditions. It may ease pain, lessen the need for drugs, stop or slow progression of a condition, or even lengthen life expectancy. Even for those in ill health, it can provide new goals and challenges to be met, and a deep sense of satisfaction in achieving these goals.

Even though you may have one or more of these special health conditions, there are still many things, such as improving your diet and stopping smoking, that you can do to improve your

Table 3.2
Medications and Exercise

Medication type	Effect on the body	Exercise precaution
Antihypertensive		
Beta blockers	Possible dizziness and faintness Feeling of weakness Reduction in: Heart rate Blood pressure The ability of the heart muscles to contract	Use *Rate of Perceived Exertion* in addition to monitoring heart rate; lower your target heart rate Avoid isometric exercises Exhale and count out loud when exerting self
Diuretics	Dizziness and faintness Low serum potassium level Fatigue and muscle cramping Thirst and dehydration Nausea and vomiting	Do not hold muscles in a contracted state for long Drink before, during, and after exercise Movements should be done slowly so as not to lose balance.
Vasodilators	Dizziness and faintness Feeling of weakness	Monitor the heart rate
Antiarrhythmic		
Digitalis- quinidine	Nausea Dizziness Headaches Drowsiness	Avoid isometric exercises Person should be constantly monitored Avoid vigorous and sustained exercise
Antiparkinsonism		
Antidepressives	Fatigue and weakness	Do gentle exercise and rhythmic activities
Dopaminergics	Appetite stimulation	
Anticholinergics	Appetite depression	

(continued)

Table 3.2. (Continued)

Medication type	Effect on the body	Exercise precaution
Antiparkinsonism (continued)		
Antihistamines	Dizziness Impairment of sweating and body cooling Blurred vision	
Antiarthritic agents		
Anti-inflammatory aspirin	Stomach irritation Swollen ankles	Avoid bouncy and jerky movements Avoid joint strain
Corticosteroids	Weight gain Gastrointestinal problems	Avoid placing body in positions that cause nausea
Psychotropic		
Sedatives	Lack of motivation	Use caution in exercises involving walking, balancing, and maintaining an upright stance
Anticonvulsants	Depression and confusion	
Antianxiety agents	Dizziness	
	Ataxia	
Antipsychotic agents	Fatigue and weakness Problem with involuntary movements, rigidity, and muscle tremors Dizziness and vertigo; disorientation in space	Use caution with exercises in which you risk falling Chair and floor exercises are more suitable
Antihistamine/ decongestants	Fatigue and weakness Appetite stimulation	Watch balance Drink fluids
Barbiturates	Possible urinary incontinence Induction of sleep Possibly habit forming Possible reduction of levels of medication in body	Do "Kegel exercises"

[a]From Fletcher (1892), Gaeta and Gaetano (1977), Piscopo (1985), Rowe and Besdine (1982), and Shepherd (1978).

general health. The following chapters will provide more ideas that will enhance your healthier lifestyle.

BIBLIOGRAPHY

References

Fletcher, G. F., 1982, *Exercise in the Practice of Medicine*, Mount Kisco, NY, Futura Publishing.

Gaeta, M. J., and Gaetano, R. J., 1977, *The Elderly: Their Health and the Drugs in Their Lives*, Dubuque, IA, Kendall Hunt Publishers.

Piscopo, J., 1985, *Fitness and Aging*, New York, John Wiley & Sons.

Rowe, J. W., and Besdine, R. W., 1982, Drug therapy, in: Rowe, J. W., Besdine, R. E., eds., *Health and Disease in Old Age*, Boston, Little, Brown & Company.

Shepherd, R. J., 1989, *Physical Activity and the Aging*, 2nd ed., Rockville, MD, Aspen Publishing.

Smith, E. L., and Surfass, R. C., eds, 1981, *Exercise and Aging: The Scientific Basis*, Hillside, NJ, Enslow Publishing.

Van Camp, S. P., and Boyer, J. L., 1989, Cardiovascular aspects of aging, *The Physician and Sportsmedicine* 17(4):121–122, 125, 128–130.

Suggested Readings and Resources

Alzheimers

Alzheimer's Disease and Related Disorders Association, Inc., 70 East Lake Street, Chicago, Illinois 60601-5997. Telephone: 1(800)621-0379.

Alzheimer's Disease Research, 15825 Shady Grove Road, Suite 140, Rockville, MD 20850. Telephone: (301) 948-3244.

Glickstein, J. K., 1988, *Therapeutic, Interventions in Alzheimer's Disease*, Rockville, MD, Aspen Publishers, Inc.

Kiely, M. A., 1985, Alzheimer's disease: making the most of the time that's left, *RN* 48(3):34–41.

Mace, N. L., and Rabins, P. V., 1981, *The 36-Hour Day*, Baltimore, The John Hopkins University Press.

Pluckhan, M. L., 1986, Alzheimer's disease: helping the patient's family, *Nursing '86*, **16**(11):62–64.

Arthritis

Arthritis Foundation, 3400 Peachtree Road, N.E., Atlanta, GA 30326.
Arthritis Today, magazine published by the Arthritis Foundation, Inc., 1314 Spring St., N. W., Atlanta, GA 30309.

American Heart Association

National Center, 7320 Greenville Avenue, Dallas, TX 75231.
They publish many free pamphlets such as "An Older Person's Guide to Cardio-vascular Health."

Incontinence

Britton, B., and Kiesling, S., 1986, The little muscle that matters, *American Health: Fitness of Body and Mind*, **5**(7):59-61.
Burgio, K. L., Pearce, K. L., Lucco, A. J., 1989, *Staying Dry: A Practical Guide to Bladder Control*, Baltimore, The Johns Hopkins University Press.
"Resource Guide of Continence Aids and Services," available from Help for Incontinent People (HIP) P.O. Box 544, Union, SC 29739.

Osteoporosis

Birge, S. J., and Dalsky, G., 1988, The role of exercise in preventing osteoporosis, *Public Health Reports Supplement*, September–October, pp. 54–58.
Dalsky, G. P., 1990, Effect of exercise on bone: Permissive influence of estrogen and calcium, *Medicine and Science in Sports and Exercise* **22**(3):281–285.
Drinkwater, B. L., 1986, Osteoporosis and the female masters athlete, in Sutton, J. A., and Brock, R. M., eds., *Sports Medicine for the Mature Athlete*, Indianapolis, IN, Benchmark Press, pp. 353–359.
Harrison, J. E., and Chow, A., 1990, Discussion: Exercise, fitness, osteoarthritis, and osteoporosis, in: Bouchard, C., Shepherd, R. J., Stevens, T., Sutton, J. R., and McPherson, B. D., eds., *Exercise, Fitness and Health: A Consensus of Current Knowledge*, Champaign, IL, Human Kinetics Publishers, pp. 529–532.

Munnings, F., 1988, Exercise and estrogen in women's health: getting a clearer picture, *The Physician and Sportsmedicine* **16**(5):152–158, 160–161.

New findings to keeping bones strong, 1990, *Running and Fitness* **8**(9):4–5.

Rikli, R. E., and McManis, B. G., 1990, Effects of exercise on bone mineral content in postmenopausal women, *Research Quarterly for Exercise and Sport* **61**(3): 243–249.

Smith E. L., 1982, Exercise for prevention of osteoporosis: a review, *The Physician and Sportsmedicine* **10**(3):72–75, 78–79, 83, 158.

Smith E. L., and Gilligan, C., 1989, Osteoporosis, bone mineral, and exercise, in: Spirduso, W. W., and Eckert, H., eds. *Physical Activity and Aging: the Academy Papers of the American Academy of Physical Education*, Champaign, IL, Human Kinetics Publishers, Inc., pp. 107-119.

Smith, E. L., Raab, D., Zook, S., and Giligan, C., 1989, Bone changes with aging and exercise, in: Harris, A., and Harris, S., eds., *Physical Activity, Aging and Sports*, Vol. 1, Albany, NY, Center for the Study of Aging, pp. 287–294.

General

Wolfe, S., 1988, *Worst Pills, Best Pills: The Older Adult's Guide To Avoiding Drug-Induced Death or Illness*, New York, Pantheon.

CHAPTER 4

Your Lifestyle and Exercise

Health and good humor are to the human body
like sunshine to vegetation.

Massillon

No part of the body or mind acts alone; each is woven into the other to create the whole person that is you: a single entity with many facets, talents, and needs. Situations, opportunities, our health, and our needs all may change as we go through life. We move, change homes, lose old friends and make new ones, lose weight, and gain weight. It is important then, as we age, to be prepared for changes. That way, we can better meet the needs and seize the opportunities that will help us gain the greatest possible amount of both good health and good humor, the "sunshine" of life.

YOUR LIFESTYLE

As you plan your exercise program, think about your whole self and remember that many factors other than your physical condition have an impact on you as you exercise, and that all of them play a role in your physical and mental fitness. These factors include your nutritional needs, your sleep needs and patterns, how you handle stress, and your exercise environment. Think of yourself as a total person as you begin your plan to create a healthier you. And remember that when we enjoy good health, in both body and spirit, our sense of well-being will grow and flourish.

Nutrition

Good nutrition involves practicing healthy eating habits throughout our lives (although it is never too late to begin). A healthy diet is one that provides all the essential nutrients: protein, carbohydrates, fats, vitamins, minerals, and water. Our overall well-being and the way our body functions are tied inextricably to our diet, as is our energy level and our physical appearance. Good nutrition can help us to look good and, better yet, to feel well.

We obtain our essential nutrients from the Four Basic Food Groups—the ones we've been hearing about since childhood. These are: (1) the milk group, (2) the meat and fish group, (3) the fruit and vegetable group, and (4) the grain group (breads and cereals).

In order to maintain a healthy nutritional plan, we should select foods from each of these groups every day. How we select our foods from within the four groups is also important, however, if we are to gain the greatest possible nutritional benefits from them. The Center for Science in the Public Interest, a nonprofit organization, has issued "The Basic Four, Revisited," which goes a step beyond merely advising that we eat the basic four food groups. It also recommends what to eat within those groups to get the maximum nutritional value from our diet. (For example, a fresh apple rather than applesauce provides more fiber and avoids the extra salt and sugar that may be added to the applesauce during the canning process.) This organization also publishes the monthly *Nutrition Action Newsletter*, which offers special rates to students and senior citizens. The address for ordering the magazine and posters can be found in the Resources Section.

In general, when planning menus we should keep in mind *Nutrition and Your Health—Dietary Guidelines for Americans*, (Department of Health and Human Services, 1986):

- Eat a variety of foods.
- Maintain a desirable weight.
- Avoid too much fat, saturated fat, and cholesterol.
- Eat foods with adequate starch and fiber.
- Avoid too much sugar.
- Avoid too much sodium.
- If you drink alcohol, do so in moderation.

In fact, moderation and variety are key words when it comes to choosing a healthy diet. Beware of food fads that promise to cure all of your ills and replace them with the vigor of a 25-year-old. Also, be wary of so-called "health foods," which have become a big and lucrative business in the past few years. Processed convenience "health" and "natural" foods are expensive for one thing, and they are not necessarily nutritious. Remember that such true health foods as fresh vegetables, dried fruits, whole-grain flours, and cereals with the least amounts of chemical additives are generally available at your local grocery store or supermarket, and usually at prices much lower than specialty or health-food stores. Read the labels carefully, compare prices and ingredients, and concentrate on fresh, nonprocessed foods.

Water is also necessary for maintaining a healthy body. When exercising, fluid intake should be increased to accomodate the requirements of increased blood circulation to the muscles and to replace the fluid that is lost as a result of sweating. For awhile, many exercise enthusiasts drank flavored and sweetened commercial products to replenish the lost fluids. Now, however, research has shown that good, pure water works just as well. If you drink bottled water, it is best to avoid those brands with a sodium content higher than 60 mg per liter. Again, read the label carefully.

Pain Control

Pain is something that is present in the lives of many people. Pain is a warning signal from the body that tells us to be aware and to do something for the body. Many people live with chronic and continuous pain, according to Bonnie Prudden, fitness teacher and developer of a promising technique of pain relief called myotherapy. This simple system focuses on the trigger points that cause muscles to go into spasm and explains how to detect these tender spots and to erase the pain by applying pressure to them. Myotherapy treats all of the possible trigger points in a given area. And there can be dozens, different in each person and resulting from a variety of lifelong events including childhood accidents, diseases, poor posture, and stress.

Myotherapy (myo = muscle) works on the muscles, and since roughly 95% of pain is muscular in origin, the technique provides a simple, safe alternative to drugs for a great many types of pain, including headache, backache, sports-related pain or that caused by overexertion, and the pain associated with arthritis and bursitis.

Although older people are said to suffer more aches and pains than younger people, Ms. Prudden's system of searching out sore spots and erasing them may provide relief from many of these nonorganic hurts. Her book, *Pain Erasure The Bonnie Prudden Way*, is filled with numerous, easy-to-understand diagrams, charts, and photographs to serve as guides.

Acupuncture/Acupressure

Acupuncture, which originated in China 2400 years ago, is another way to alleviate pain. It is one of the world's oldest medical treatments, and has become one of the fastest growing healthcare methods in the United States. It is based on the theory of "Ji," which is the flow of the life force or body energy through the body. This concept also appears in yoga where it is called "prana," which is the term for "life force" in the language of Sanskrit. There are 14 main, invisible pathways, called meridians, in the body. Disease or pain can develop when there is a blockage along these meridians. By stimulating one of the 365 points along the meridians (either by inserting needles, applying the modern device of electrical current similar to ultrasound, or using acupressure), the "Ji" is stimulated.

Acupuncture as a means of pain control has been widely studied by Dr. Ji-Shen Han, Chairman of the Department of Physiology and Director of the Neuroscience Research Center at Beijing Medical University and author of the book, *Neurochemical Basis of Pain Relief by Acupuncture*. In 1965 and 1966, he conducted research on 66 human subjects. He resumed his research on rats and rabbits following the Cultural Revolution in 1972 and it is continuing to the present. His early research found that levels of the neurotransmitter serotonin rose following acupuncture, resulting in a pain-killing effect on the subject. Acupuncture is also used in China as a form of anesthesia during surgery and childbirth. In the United States it is used to assist people in breaking addictive habits such as the use of drugs, smoking, and eating disorders. Good results have also been reported in treating migraine headaches, whiplash, osteoarthritis, and musculoskeletal problems of the lower back, shoulders, and knees. It is possible to learn to apply self pressure to the acupuncture sites for relief of various ailments (Figs. 4.1 to 4.3).

The use of acupuncture techniques can be beneficial to the older adult in many ways. It certainly cannot be harmful or cause harmful side effects as drugs may often do. It cannot cure cancer or other long term, debilitating diseases, but it can help ease the pain. It is recommended that a person first see a physician before being referred for acupuncture or acupressure treatment. A list of those who are licensed to practice acupuncture and the states that allow acupuncture is available through the organizations listed in the Resources.

Sleep

An adequate amount of sleep is necessary to maintain the energy required for an exercise program. However, what is considered adequate may vary at different ages and among different individuals. In general, older people seem to require less sleep, although some researchers believe that in actuality older people sleep less because they do not sleep as well. Whatever the theories, a good night's sleep for any individual is that amount that allows him or her to feel rested the next day.

Many older persons suffer from insomnia, either occasionally or chronically. There may be a number of reasons for these sleep disturbances, including physical ailments, medications, financial or psychological worries, and traumatic life events. One of the most important causes, however, is inactivity. The lifestyle of Americans in general is becoming more sedentary, and as we grow older this may become even more true. It has been shown that regular exercise improves sleep because it refreshes and relaxes, clears the mind, and encourages good sleep.

Instructions for Locating Sites

1. Concentration, Memory point: Located on a line straight up from the nose, over the top of the head in a hollow just behind the crown.

2. Nasal congestion point: Run finger up the side of the nose until it reaches the top of a triangle of cartilage.

3. Toothache point: Located in the corner of the jaw and found by running finger up towards ear (approximately 1 inch) until it falls in hollow.

4. Cough and asthma points : 2 points- Located just over and behind the bone in the hollow of the throat. 2nd point on midline of the body even with the level of the nipples.

5. Stomach ache point: Located on the midline of the front of the body halfway between the bottom of the sternum and the navel.

6. Water retention and menstrual pain/ problems: Located on the line going down the leg from the medial side of the kneecap, approximately 5 fingers distance from the kneecap and over the round top of the bone.

7. Water retention and menstrual pain/ problems: Located up from the inside of the ankle bone 4 fingers distance and back from the shinbone approximately 1/2 to 3/4 inch.

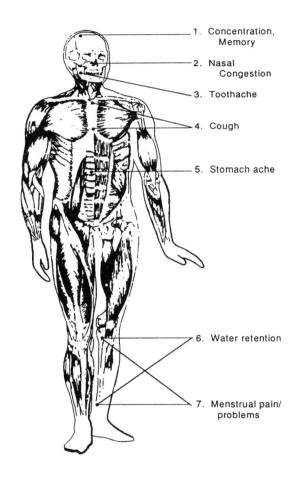

1. Concentration, Memory
2. Nasal Congestion
3. Toothache
4. Cough
5. Stomach ache
6. Water retention
7. Menstrual pain/ problems

Figure 4.1. Acupressure for front of body. From *Hatha Yoga: Developing the Body, Mind and Inner Self,* by DeeAnn Birkel, Eddie Bowers Publishing, Inc., Dubuque, Iowa. Reprinted with permission.

Instructions for Locating Sites

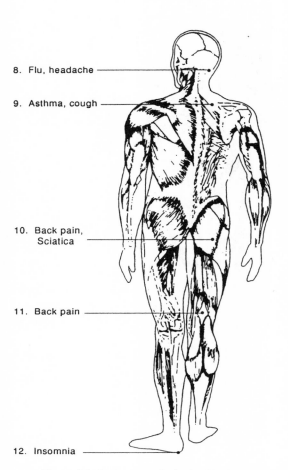

8. Flu, headache

9. Asthma, cough

10. Back pain, Sciatica

11. Back pain

12. Insomnia

8. Flu and Headache point: Located in a hollow where the skull meets the neck muscles on the back of the head. This point will be very sore if you are coming down with the flu or a cold.

9. Asthma and cough points (3 points each side): Located approximately 1 inch, 1 1/2 inch and 2 inches out from the 1st thoracic vertebrae which is at the level of the shoulders.

10. Back pain and sciatica point: Located just lateral to the center of each buttock. You will be able to tell when you have located this point because it gives a strong reaction.

11. Back pain point: Located on the crease in the center of the back of the knee and is easiest to find and apply pressure to while the knee is bent.

12. Insomnia point: In the center of the heel on the bottom of the foot.

Figure 4.2. Acupressure for back of body. From *Hatha Yoga: Developing with Body, Mind and Inner Self,* by DeeAnn Birkel, Eddie Bowers Publishing, Inc., Dubuque, Iowa. Reprinted with permission.

Instructions for Locating Sites

13. Insomnia point: Located just over the bone on crease of the wrist on a line running straight up the arm from the little finger.

14. Nausea, morning and carsickness point: Located on the inside of the wrist between the middle tendons and up the distance found by placing 4 fingers close together on the wrist crease.

15. Nosebleed point: Located on the outside corner of thumbnail. It is most effective to hold a burning stick of incense near the site to stop bleeding.

16. Headache and toothache point: Located at the top of the fleshy mound found by bringing thumb next to hand. Press down on the top of the crease nearest wrist, and inward towards the fingers, while index finger is pressing up from the bottom. This gives a strong reaction.

17. Hiccups point: Located on the ear where the top part curves in and flattens out.

18. Headache, hangover point: Located on the ear lobe.

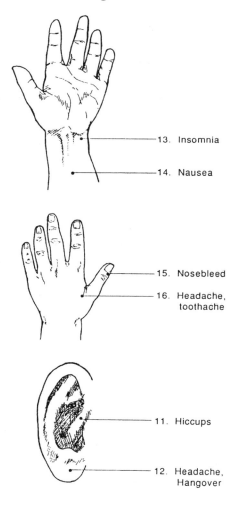

13. Insomnia

14. Nausea

15. Nosebleed

16. Headache, toothache

11. Hiccups

12. Headache, Hangover

Drawings by Lydia Gerbig, a Ball State University graduate.

Figure 4.3. Accupressure for hand and ear. From *Hatha Yoga: Developing the Body, Mind and Inner Self,* by DeeAnn Birkel, Eddie Bowers Publishing, Inc., Dubuque, Iowa. Reprinted with permission.

Stress

In these fast-paced times, stress and anxiety trouble many people, and older people are certainly no exception. In fact, depression and suicide, two unfortunate outcomes of stress, are not uncommon among the older population. But feeling "down" is not inevitable. Research has proven that being involved in exercise greatly reduces the impact that stress has on our health and life.

We react to stress in many ways; to discover how you respond, do the questionnaire in Fig. 4.4. This questionnaire was developed by Merrill F. Raber and George Dyck. The questionnaire helps pinpoint your reactions to stressful situations. If some of your responses fall in the "need to improve" category you may want to incorporate stress-reducing activities into the new healthier lifestyle that you are planning for yourself. In a few weeks repeat this quiz and write your answers with a different color of ink so you can easily see any changes.

As we go through life, our stressors change. It is important to remember that both good and bad things cause stress. The Holmes and Rahe Social Readjustment Rating Scale, developed in 1967, measures the major events in life and assigns points to each event. A glance at this scale (see Appendix E) will help you identify sources of stress in your own life.

As with any kind of fitness program, your program to reduce stress should begin with an activity you enjoy. It is generally accepted that physical activity is one of the best means of easing tension and reducing the amount of stress you feel. But a physical activity need not be rigorous to be stress-relieving. It may be as simple as lying still for a few moments and relaxing each of your muscles, one by one, beginning with your head and neck and moving on down your body and ending with your feet and toes. Or you may choose a game or sport you particularly like or go for a brisk walk with a friend. All of these activities can calm and refresh you and help you to cope with the stress, both good and bad, that is a part of most lives today.

Place a check in the appropriate column. Try to be completely honest.	I do well (5 pts)	I'm average (3 pts)	Need to improve (1 pt)
1. "Owning" my own stress (not blaming others).	___	___	___
2. Knowing my level of optimum stress (the level of stress that allows me to do my best without becoming destructive).	___	___	___
3. Balancing work and play (scheduling time for play).	___	___	___
4. Loafing more (learning to do nothing at times and feel okay about it).	___	___	___
5. Getting enough sleep and rest rather than ending up with what is left over at the end of the day (scheduling adequate sleep).	___	___	___
6. Refusing to take on more than I can handle (learning to say no).	___	___	___
7. Working off tension (hard physical effort on a regular basis).	___	___	___
8. Setting realistic goals (goals that can be achieved within a reasonable time frame).	___	___	___
9. Practicing relaxation (meditating with music or biofeedback).	___	___	___
10. Slowing down (taking pleasure in every moment rather than rushing through life).	___	___	___
11. Putting emphasis on being rather than doing (being a person others like to be around is more important than "doing" many activities).	___	___	___
12. Managing my time, including planning for time alone (setting priorities and doing those things that are most important).	___	___	___
13. Planning regular recreation (recreation is a complete change of pace and something that is fun to do).	___	___	___

(continued)

Figure 4.4. Stress Releases and Safety Valves. Reprinted with permission from M. Raber and G. Dyck, *Mental Fitness: A Guide to Emotional Health*, pp. 23–24, Crisp Publications, Inc., 95 First Street, Los Altos, Calif. 94022.

14. Having a physical fitness program (having a   ____   ____   ____
    specific plan for strenuous exercise).
15. Avoiding too much caffeine (limiting coffee   ____   ____   ____
    and cola drinks).
16. Emphasizing good nutrition in diet (learning   ____   ____   ____
    about nutrition and avoiding junk foods.)
17. Avoiding alcohol or other chemicals to deal   ____   ____   ____
    with pressure (dependency on alcohol or
    drugs deals with symptoms rather than the
    problem).
18. Avoiding emotional "overload" (taking on   ____   ____   ____
    problems of others when you are under
    stress is destructive).
19. Selecting emotional "investments" more   ____   ____   ____
    carefully (of things we can get involved with
    that call for emotional involvement it is nec-
    essary to choose carefully).
20. Giving and accepting positive "strokes" (be-   ____   ____   ____
    ing able to express positive things to others
    and to receive positive comments in return
    is an achievement).
21. Talking out troubles and getting professional   ____   ____   ____
    help if needed (being willing to seek help is
    a sign of strength rather than weakness).

To Score Yourself

If you scored between 21 and 50, there are several areas you need to develop to better release your stress. It might be a good idea to discuss some of your answers with a counselor or close friend.

If you scored between 51 and 75, you have discovered a variety of ways to deal effectively with stress. Make a note of those items you checked "need to improve" and work on strategies to help you move to the "I'm Average" box.

If your score was 75 or greater—congratulations. You apparently have found some excellent ways to deal with frustration and the complexities of life. Stay alert to protect the valuable skills you have acquired.

Figure 4.4. (continued)

Smoking

Smoking has a negative impact on the body at any time, but it also complicates the exercise plan. The body needs oxygen in every cell to stay alive and functioning, and the muscle cells demand even more oxygen when they are involved in exercise. Smoking greatly inhibits the oxygen transport system of the body. The lungs actually become diseased as a result of the disappearance of the cilia which filter the pollutants in the air we breathe. Mucus is then formed as a protective measure, but it eventually becomes trapped in the lungs and causes "smoker's cough." Smoking is also a factor in the development of emphysema, a disease that destroys the elasticity of the lungs and their ability to properly inhale and exhale the air. All of these losses mean that less oxygen comes into the body and this in turn lessens our ability to undertake physical activities and perform routine tasks.

The nicotine in cigarettes causes the heart to work harder, the pulse rate to increase, the blood pressure to increase, and the air passages of the lungs to narrow, thus producing a reduction in the oxygen exchange. The result is less oxygen available to the heart and muscles. In addition, smoking produces carbon monoxide in the bloodstream. Carbon monoxide binds more easily with hemoglobin (which is the major oxygen-carrying component of the red blood cells) than oxygen does. As a result, still less oxygen is available to the body.

Both the American Heart Association and the American Cancer Society have conducted and funded research on the adverse effects of smoking, and their findings are dramatic. Smokers are twice as likely to die from heart diseases as nonsmokers, and one of five cancer deaths is due to smoking. Research indicates that cancers caused by smoking are 100% preventable.

Even if you are a long-time smoker, it is not too late to quit, and there are almost immediate health benefits. Within 20 min of your last cigarette your blood pressure and pulse rate drop. Within

8 hr of your last smoke the carbon monoxide level in your body will drop to normal; this allows the oxygen level to increase—and it really does! Within only two weeks the body's circulation improves, walking becomes easier, and lung function increases up to 30%. From one to nine months after you quit, the mucus problem improves and the smoker's cough lessens as a result of the re-growth of the cilia in the lungs. When you quit smoking you will have much more energy available to enjoy to the fullest the benefits of your exercise. Many older people, who began smoking when it was not recognized as a health hazard, have rid themselves of the habit and replaced it with the positive experience of exercise and activity. You can do it too.

CHOOSING THE APPROPRIATE ATTIRE

As you adopt a new more active lifestyle, you may want to purchase some new clothing for exercise. This does not mean breaking your budget on the latest in fitness fashions from health clubs and spas, but rather choosing clothing and shoes that will permit you to exercise comfortably, safely, and with self-confidence. It is nice to feel that you look good as you exercise, but it is even more important to know that your exercise attire will permit you the comfort and freedom to gain the maximum benefits from your workout.

Clothing

The most important thing to remember when choosing clothing is to dress appropriately for the temperature, taking into consideration whether you are exercising inside or outdoors. You do not want to be too warm, so wearing clothing in layers is a good idea. Soft, loose clothing lets you move comfortably. There are many fabric types to choose from, including cotton, Lycra, nylon, spandex, and polypropylene. Cotton absorbs the body's moisture better than synthetic fabrics do and it allows the body to "breathe." Don't wear heavy support garments like girdles because they inhibit circulation and strengthening of the muscles. Some people may find it necessary to wear support hose because of problems with varicose veins. If you do, be careful not to become overheated, because support hose inhibit the body's cooling process by means of evaporation of sweat on the surface of the skin. Women should always wear a bra that gives good support, and men should wear an athletic supporter.

Soft, fleece "warm-up" suits of matching pants and top or jacket are becoming more popular with all age groups and both sexes because of their wonderful comfort. Do not buy a rubber sweat suit, because there have been deaths associated with these. Nylon sweat suits zipped up and fitting tight at the wrists and ankles have also been known to cause death on a hot, humid day.

In general, clothing should fit comfortably and be loose enough to allow freedom of movement without confinement or embarrassment to the wearer. When exercising in the cold, it is important to wear a hat and gloves, since it has been found that 75–85% of the body's heat is lost through the head and hands. The rest of the clothing should be in layers, preferably with one layer of wool. The new polypropylene "warm-up" suits are expensive but provide warmth and protection from the cold and dampness.

We'll talk more about exercising in extreme heat or cold following the section on footwear.

Footwear

Footwear is the most important item of clothing to consider if you are planning to walk or to do a form of low-impact aerobics. The ideal shoe for walking should provide support and absorb force. Always wear a sock or footlet for all forms of exercise to prevent blisters.

The sole of a walking shoe generally is thinner and softer than that of other sport shoes, and it should flex easily as your foot bends. The soles are flatter than those of running shoes, which have lugs or other traction surfaces that may trip you during walking. The sole of a good walking shoe curves up at the toe to allow for the rolling motion your foot makes when you walk. The toe box (the part that encloses your toes) should be large enough to allow space for the toes to spread. The arch should be firm and give you good support, but it should not be higher than what you are currently wearing.

The heel should be reinforced to help prevent a natural tendency of the ankle to pronate, or twist inward, when the heel strikes the ground. This twisting action can cause leg and lower back injuries as well as sore feet. The heel counter should extend further toward the toe than it does in running shoes. The upper part of the shoe can be of either nylon, suede, or leather. If you live in a warm climate nylon is cooler, especially the new nylon mesh. Leather is warmer, molds to the shape of the foot, and can be waterproofed for wearing in the winter. Suede is good because it has the benefits of leather but is somewhat lighter.

For cycling, either on an exercise cycle or a bicycle, you need a shoe that has cushioning over the midsole. The shoes worn for race-cycling are different and will not be discussed here. Refer to a cycling book if you are interested in that activity.

If you want to dance, the type of dancing you will be doing determines the choice of a shoe. If you choose to do low-impact aerobic dance, which is becoming increasingly popular, consider the following points when selecting a shoe for this activity:

1. *Sole.* You must have shoes that are designed to minimize stress to the knees, lower legs, ankles, and feet. The sole

should also be very flexible, so fold the shoe to see if the toe can fit into the heel. In addition, the sole should not have lugs like running shoes, because these can stick to the floor and may trip you. The soles should have lines, however, to provide some traction.

2. *Heel Box.* In aerobic dance, there is a great deal of lateral (sideways) movement, and the ankles are better supported if the heel box is extra firm.

3. *Lacing.* The lacing should be spaced close together to provide more support for the lateral movement.

4. *Uppers.* Nylon is cooler, but leather and suede wear longer. A combination is good, with the leather along the toes where there is more stress on the shoe.

For folk, square, or social dancing, the shoe should have a 1–1½ inch heel and should also lace or have a strap for stability. The sole should be leather, which allows the foot to pivot and slide. Do not do these dance activities in a shoe with a rubber sole because it may stick and cause you to trip and pull a muscle.

Since your main expense in beginning an exercise program will probably be your shoe, you should do some looking and comparison shopping before you buy. Don't skimp and choose footwear that does not meet the requirements discussed. Shop around using the checklist in Fig. 4.5 to get the best buy for your needs and money. Take a copy of the checklist with you when you shop for a shoe (see Appendix F).

It is not necessary to have the most expensive shoe on the market; that may not be the best one for you. However, don't settle for a shoe that does not meet your needs just to save money. Give this some serious thought and planning, and try on several shoes before you make your final purchase.

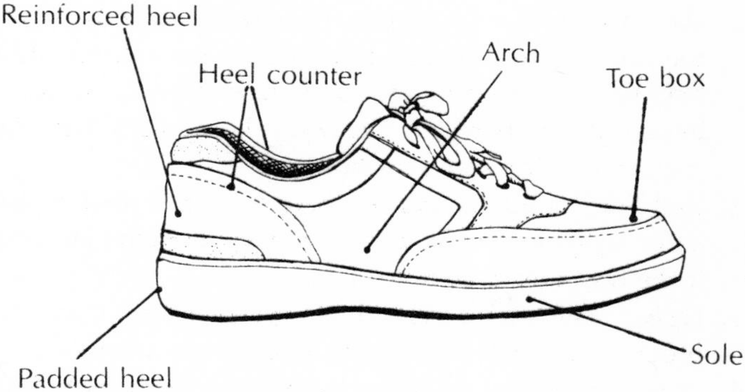

Figure 4.5. Checklist for shoe purchase.

1. I want a shoe for (list activity) _____
2. The shoe has laces   Yes _____   No _____
3. The sole flexes   Yes _____   No _____
4. The sole provides adequate traction   Yes _____   No _____
5. The arch fits my foot   Yes _____   No _____
6. The arch has removable inner support   Yes _____   No _____
7. The toe box does not crowd my toes   Yes _____   No _____
8. The uppers are: Nylon _____
                    Nylon mesh _____
                    Leather _____
9. Cost and name
   a _____
   b _____
   c _____

WEATHER

Be aware of the weather. In summer, avoid walking or cycling outside in the heat of day. In winter, be sure you are dressed properly, and be especially careful to keep your hands and head covered and your feet warm. Although exercise at cooler temperatures is invigorating it is best in colder weather to wait until afternoon to exercise out of doors. Be careful to avoid icy or unsafe surfaces. Wearing light-colored clothing in hot weather will help you stay comfortable as you exercise, and a light hat will also keep you cooler. Be sure to drink plenty of water to prevent dehydration. Many people prefer to walk in shopping malls to avoid the extremes in the weather. This permits exercise in a stable environment all year round. Please refer to Fig. 4.6 and Table 4.1 as you make your plans for exercise in various kinds of weather and climates. A basic rule would be to avoid being out in extreme heat combined with high humidity and extreme cold combined with wind, ice, or snow.

SUMMARY

Now that you have examined the various aspects of your lifestyle and looked at the effect they will have on you as you exercise, it is time to move on to some practical guidelines, techniques, and safety tips as well as a step-by-step plan to follow each time you exercise. Exercise is one of the best things you can do for your health. Keeping these things in mind will help you to get the most from your exercise program.

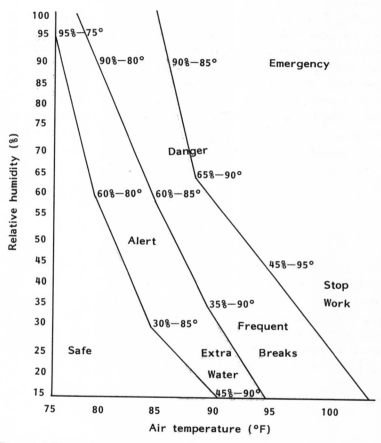

Figure 4.6. Heat–safety index. From Ball State University Weather Station, Department of Geography, Muncie, Indiana. Reprinted with permission.

Table 4.1
Wind-Chill Factor[a,b]

| Wind speed | | Actual thermometer reading (°F) | | | | | | | | | | |
Knots	mph	50	40	30	20	10	0	-10	-20	-30	-40	-50
		Equivalent temperature (°F)										
Calm		50	40	30	20	10	0	-10	-20	-30	-40	-50
4	5	48	37	27	16	6	-5	-15	-26	-36	-47	-57
9	10	40	28	16	4	-9	-21	-33	-46	-58	-70	-83
13	15	36	22	9	-5	-18	-36	-45	-58	-72	-85	-99
17	20	32	18	4	-10	-25	-39	-53	-67	-82	-96	-110
22	25	30	16	0	-15	-29	-44	-59	-74	-88	-104	-118
26	30	28	23	-2	-18	-33	-48	-63	-79	-84	-109	-125
30	35	21	11	-4	-20	-35	-49	-67	-82	-96	-113	-129
35	40	26	10	-6	-21	-37	-53	-69	-85	-100	-116	-132

Wind speeds greater than 40 have little additional effect

Little danger
(for properly clothed person)

Increasing danger

Great danger

[a]This is an index of the cooling power of the wind. It is expressed in terms of the equivalent temperature without wind. The wind-chill index describes the cooling effect of any combination of temperature and winds.

[b]Source: Ball State University Weather Station, Department of Geography, Muncie, Indiana.

BIBLIOGRAPHY

References

Han, J. S., 1973–1987, *Neurochemical Basis of Pain Relief by Acupuncture*, collection of papers, 1973–1987, Beijing Medical School.

Holmes, T. H., and Rahe, R. H., 1967, The Social Readjustment Scale, *Journal of Psychosomatic Research* **11**:213–218.

Raber, M. F., and Dyck, G., 1987, *Mental Fitness: A Guide to Emotional Health*, Crisp Publications, Inc., Los Altos, CA.

United States Department of Health and Human Services, 1986, *Nutrition and Your Health—Dietary Guidelines for Americans*, United States Department of Health and Human Services, Washington, DC.

Suggested Reading

Benfante, R., 1990, Keeping older hearts healthy, *Prevention* **42**:16–18.

Brady, S. R., 1987, Acupuncture and Me, *Good Housekeeping* **205**(2):58–62.

Coleman, E., 1985, Dietary goals for the active older person, *Sports Medicine Digest* **7**(9):7.

Faber, W. J., and Walker, M, 1990, *Pain Go Away*, Mountain View, CA, ISHI Press International.

Greeley, A., 1990, Nutrition and the elderly, *FDA Consumer* **24**:24–28.

Kapp, M. B., 1990, Empowering the elderly: dignity and health, *Current* **319**:10–13.

Manaka, Y., 1972, *Layman's Guide to Acupuncture*, Rutland VT, Charles E. Tuttel Publisher.

Maxwell, R. B., 1990, AARP 90s goal—good health for all, *Modern Maturity* **33**:10–11.

Poppy, J., 1989, Thirty years of fortitude, *Esquire* **112**:83–85.

Prudden, B., 1977, *Pain Erasure the Bonnie Prudden Way*, New York, M. Evans & Company, Inc.

Rizzler, C. A., 1990, Foods that fight aging, *Readers Digest* **137**:13–14.

Rodale, R., 1990, Radical regeneration, *Prevention* **42**:30–32.

Rodarmor, W., 1986, Acupuncture comes of age in America, *Yoga Journal*, **67**:26–29, 64.

Rubenstein, C., 1990, Here's to your health, *New Choices for the Best Years* **30**:35–39.

Stark, E., 1989, Who stays fit, *Psychology Today* **23**:73.

Stein, D., 1988, Interview: Ji-Sheng Han, *OMNI Magazine* **10**:81–85, 102.

Tiidus, P., Shephard, R. J., and Montelpare, W., 1989, Overall intake of energy and key nutrients: data for middle-aged and older middle-class adults, *Canadian Journal of Sport Sciences* **14**(3):173–177.

Update on acupuncture, 1986, *Changing Times* **40**(9):12–13.

Vega, C., 1987, Nutrition for active seniors, *Dance Exercise Today* **5**(7):51–54.

Wagner, L., and Klein, R. M., 1989, The acupressure face-lift, *New Age Journal* **6**(2):29–34.

Walford, R. L., 1986, *The 120-Year Diet*, New York, Simon and Schuster.

Resources

Books

Brody, J., 1981, *Jane Brody's Nutrition Book*, New York, W.W. Norton & Company.

Newsletters

Nutrition Action Health Newsletter, Center for Science in the Public Interest, 1501 16th St. N.W., Washington, D.C. 20036.

The Johns Hopkins Medical Letter: Health After 50. The Johns Hopkins Medical Institutions, 550 North Broadway, Suite 1100, Johns Hopkins, Baltimore, MD 21205.

University of California, Berkeley Wellness Letter, Health Letter Associates, P.O. Box 420148, Palm Coast, FL 32142.

Organizations

The Traditional Acupuncture Foundation, American City Building, Suite 100, Columbia, MD 21044. Telephone (301) 997-4888.

Acupuncture Research Institute, 313 West Andrix St., Monterey Park, CA 91754.

CHAPTER 5
The Basics of Exercise

He who has health has hope, and he who has
hope has everything.

Arabian proverb

The preliminaries are over. By now you have had a complete medical examination and have gathered information about your physical status and your attitudes regarding exercise and life in general. You have identified the causes of stress in your life and have seen that exercise is an excellent way of coping with them. You have also become aware of your nutritional and clothing needs. Finally, you have measured your own individual strengths by means of a series of self-appraisal tests and have recorded the results. You are almost ready to begin exercise. But before you do, read through the following basic guidelines for exercisers.

BASIC GUIDELINES

As you begin your program of exercise, here are some simple things to do and to avoid, to help you get the most from your exercise program.

Start off Slowly

Remember that any amount of exercise, however little, is better than none at all. It is easy to be enthusiastic as you begin, but doing too much too soon is unwise. Do not try to do too many exercises or too many repetitions of the exercises you have chosen. Three to five times each will be enough to start. Do the same number of repetitions a second day, and then add one repetition each day until you are doing the desired number.

If you have previously been inactive or if it has been a number of years since you have participated in sports or practiced a regular exercise routine, be sure to start with just a short period of exercise. Five to ten minutes twice a week is a safe way to begin, adding a few more minutes each week. Eventually you will want to work up to 15 to 30 min each time, three to four times a week. If you are overweight or seriously out of shape you will probably want to precondition yourself with a program of walking or light warm-up or cool-down exercises before you begin any program of physical activity at all. After 3 to 6 weeks, having noticed improvement, you may feel like increasing the duration of your exercise program.

It is most important to exercise regularly, even if the total number of times per week is small. Try to maintain a regular schedule, but stop if you become ill, and remember to re-start at a lower level of activity. If you have persistent muscle soreness that does not go away after 1 or 2 weeks, or if you feel exceptionally fatigued, you are probably trying to exercise too hard. Cut back on your exercise routine by slowing the pace and reducing the number of repetitions of the exercise. This gives your body more time to adjust to your new regimen of physical activity. Remember that your exercise program should include stretching and flexibility exercises as well as aerobic activities such as walking, swimming, cycling, or dancing. Avoid all activities that involve jumping or pounding motions, such as vigorous aerobic dance or jogging.

Warm up and Cool down

Never fail to allow 5 to 10 min for warming up and 5 min for cooling down. (See the basic warm-up and basic cool-down routines presented in Chapter 6, pages 133 to 134.) You may not want to take the extra time, but the older you are, the more important it is to prepare your body for exercise with a warm up and then allow it to cool down afterwards. For the cool down, slow down the pace of your activity and do some of the same stretches you did for the warm up. Never neglect this important part of the exercise program and no matter how inviting it may seem, avoid taking a hot shower or sauna immediately after a strenuous workout. Since heat opens the blood vessels, which may cause circulatory collapse, you should wait at least 5 min before you take a shower, and then keep the water warm, not hot.

Monitor Your Pulse and Exertion Level

Your pulse is one of the best indicators of how your body is responding to exercise. Your heart rate is a principal means of assessing your body's performance and plays an important part in determining the level and extent of the exercise you undertake. To determine your maximum heart rate, subtract your age from 220.

Exercisers who are over 50 are generally advised to exercise at a heart rate that is 50% to 60% of their maximum heart rate, although older people can benefit from exercise at 40% of capacity done for a longer period of time. This percentage of maximum heart rate is called the target range. Table 5.1, from the American Heart Association, gives the minimum and maximum levels (target ranges) for a variety of age groups.

However, remember that this is only a general guideline. The formula for figuring your target heart rate is included in the Exercise Program Worksheet presented in Table 5.4. If your own heart rate varies greatly from the recommended target range or if you have a medical history of heart problems, consult your physician. If you experience difficulty exercising even at the minimum level, ease up and exercise less intensely but for a longer period of time.

A person who is in generally good health and has been

Table 5.1
Suggested Target Heart Rate Range[a]

Age (years)	Target zone[b] (beats per min)	Average maximum heart rate (100%)
40	90–108	180
45	87–105	175
50	85–102	170
55	82–99	165
60	80–96	160
65	77–93	155
70	75–90	150
75	72–87	145
80	70–84	140
85	67–81	135

[a]Based on recommendations by the American Heart Association.
[b]50% to 60% of maximum heart rate.

cleared for exercise by his or her physician should not have to worry about undertaking a regular exercise program. However, all people should be aware of the danger signs that may accompany exercise. (See the American Heart Association Warning Signs of a Heart Attack presented in Table 5.2.)

Excessive breathlessness or chest pain are always signals to stop the activity and call your doctor, as is any pain or discomfort in the upper neck or lower face. This fact is not so well known, so be aware that any pain in these areas is also a warning signal. No matter what your level of physical condition, it is important to be aware of how you feel after exercise. According to Dr. Charles Kuntzleman, YMCA exercise consultant who is quoted in the *Guide for Those Over 50,* by the AMA, if you are tired or short of breath for the rest of the afternoon or evening following your workout, you are most likely overexerting and should ease up. If after 2 or 3 hr you feel good, then you are probably exercising at a

Table 5.2
Warning Signs of a Heart Attack

---

1. Chest discomfort is the most significant signal of a heart attack.
   Character: Uncomfortable pressure, squeezing, fullness or tightness, aching.
   Location: Center of the chest behind the breastbone. May spread to the shoulder, neck, or arms.
   Duration: Usually lasts longer than 2 min. May come and go.
2. Other signs may include any or all of the following:
   Sweating
   Nausea
   Shortness of breath
   Weakness
3. However, be alert to the fact that:
   The pain may not be severe.
   The person may not "look poorly" or have all of the symptoms.
   Sharp, stabbing, short twinges of pain usually are not signals of a heart attack.

---

aBased on *Student Manual for Basic Life Support: Cardiopulmonary Resuscitation,* American Heart Association.

level that is right for you. "Remember," says Dr. Kuntzleman, "exercise is not supposed to leave you exhausted. It is supposed to leave you revitalized" (Kuntzleman, 1984).

Pay Attention to Perceived Exertion

The Rate of Perceived Exertion is another way to monitor your exercise session. It takes into consideration other factors beside pulse rate; for example, your energy level, how tired you felt while exercising and at the end of your exercise period, your muscular strength and flexibility level, and how hard you think you worked. It involves picking a number that reflects an exercise workout, ranging from 6 (very, very light) to 20 (very, very hard). This method is gaining in popularity and is taught to participants in cardiac rehabilitation programs as a way to monitor more thoroughly their response to the exercise session. The following chart (from Borg, 1973) presents the levels of perceived exertion (Table 5.3).

Table 5.3
Rating of Perceived Exertion[a]

6		13	Somewhat hard
7	Very, very light	14	
8		15	Hard
9	Very light	16	
10		17	Very hard
11	Fairly light	18	
12		19	Very, very hard
		20	

[a]From G. Borg, Perceived exertion: a note on history and methods, *Medicine and Science in Sports and Exercise,* **5:**90–93, 1973, © American College of Sports Medicine. Reprinted with permission.

Concentrate on Proper Breathing

Oxygen is necessary for muscles to do their work, so it is most important to keep up a steady breathing pattern throughout exercise. Do not hold your breath during exertion, but instead breathe vigorously—in through the nose and out through the mouth. Counting aloud slowly as you exhale keeps the throat open and prevents increased pressure in the blood vessels and chest, which may result in ruptured blood vessels.

Listen to Your Body

As you exercise, your body is constantly responding, telling you how you are progressing, how well you are doing. Pay attention when your body tells you to slow down or stop! Normally you will experience some tiredness or feelings of fatigue, and as you exercise you may be aware of having worked long-unused muscles and joints. This is natural and to be expected as you begin your program of more strenuous exercise and physical activity. But if you experience persistent pain, stop! Begin again at a lower level of exertion and build up gradually. Remember, if you experience chest pain, breathlessness, severe joint discomfort, or recurring muscle cramps, call your doctor. You have lived with your body for some time now, and you, perhaps better than anyone, know what is normal for your body—when things feel right and when they do not. Remember, your exercise program is intended to make you feel healthy and well. It is not an endurance contest. When your body is telling you it is not feeling up to par, slow down. With time and persistence, your body will most probably tell you it is feeling stronger and healthier.

Involve Your Mind

Your mind, along with your body, plays an important part in your physical and mental well-being. Make your mindset an integral part of your exercise routine. It helps to read articles, books, and other materials that explain the benefits of exercise and provide encouragement as you begin your own program of self-improvement. Use imagery to see yourself in a healthier state. Be realistic, of course, but practice seeing yourself standing tall, head held high, alert, with clear eyes and a smile on your face. See yourself eating a healthier diet, giving up smoking, and exercising regularly. See yourself as the best you can be, and then strive to be the person you see.

Plan for Relaxation in Your Day

Give some thought to a time for relaxation or meditation every day. Meditation can be as simple and down-to-earth as sitting quietly with your eyes closed visualizing some especially pleasant scene or place. Or allow for time alone listening to your favorite classical or instrumental music or to one of the newer recordings of soothing sounds such as rain, sea sounds, or forest noises. Anything without a strong beat or rhythm is wonderfully relaxing. Another soothing, stress-reducing practice is to lie flat on your back on the floor (or on your bed, if you prefer) with your legs slightly apart, your arms 6 to 10 in from your body with palms up, your head straight, and your eyes closed ever so lightly. Drift this way, awake and yet totally relaxed. Allow at least 10 min a day for this type of relaxation. Some people end their daily workout with a 10-min period of total relaxation. You will be amazed at how this simple practice will invigorate you and refresh you for the day ahead.

Have Fun

This may be one of the most important things to remember about exercising. Choose an activity you will truly enjoy; that way, you are most likely to stay with it, to look forward to it, and to have a good time doing it. "The biggest problem for most middle-aged adults is that they *hate* exercise, not in and of itself, but because of past associations and ideas" (Kuntzleman, 1984). Many of us would agree with Dr. Kuntzleman. For those who have memories of exercise sessions that are less than pleasant, now is the time to replace those memories with new and positive attitudes about exercise. There are so many options available and so many different and enjoyable activities to help us feel more vigorous, attractive, healthy, and, yes, even younger. The delightful thing about being an older adult is that we are free to choose exactly what we want—dancing, swimming, cycling with a companion, or walking briskly, either alone or with a friend. We can choose solitude or companionship, the hustle and bustle of a shopping mall or city park, or the quiet of a small neighborhood, or, even our own living room. No one is there to dictate how or when we must exercise.

Give some careful thought to what you would really enjoy, not what magazines, experts, or teachers say you should enjoy. Then begin to do that activity and stick with it. Don't ever forget the element of fun. An exercise routine that lacks this important ingredient is doomed to fail, perhaps not right away, but eventually. Above all, don't overload yourself with guilt if you are not a totally dedicated, enthusiastic exerciser, especially at first. Many people are not. Do recognize how important it is to strive for the healthiest state possible and, most importantly, keep it enjoyable. Set goals that are safe and attainable and then stay with the routine you have chosen. It takes awhile, perhaps several months, for you to become comfortable with your routine and to begin to really enjoy regular exercise, so promise yourself to give it a try for at least that long. If you do not give up within the first few weeks, you may find that you have improved your level of fitness and are now feeling better and more energetic than you have in years. If the routine you plan for yourself is enjoyable and geared to your own special needs and wants as an older person, you may soon find that you look forward to it eagerly.

Safety Considerations

Although exercise is one of the best things you do for your health, it is nevertheless wise to keep in mind a few special considerations that will help you avoid injury or illness while you are working out.

1. Always drink water before and after your exercise session to avoid dehydration. Be especially concerned about this in summer and in hot climates.
2. Be aware of the weather. In the summer, avoid walking or cycling outside in the heat of the day. If you are in doubt about how much is too much, refer to the chart of air temperature and humidity given in Fig. 4.6. In the winter, it is best to wait until later in the day to exercise outdoors.
3. Walk on sidewalks whenever possible. If you must walk in the street or road, walk facing the traffic and wear bright clothing so that you are highly visible. At dusk or night-time wear reflective clothing.
4. Take your pulse at the beginning, halfway through, and at the end of your exercise period. (If you have questions about how to do this, refer to Fig. 2.2, for locating pulse at wrist and neck.) Remember, you either count for 10 sec and multiply by 6, or count for 6 sec and add a zero to get your estimated pulse rate for 1 min.

An exercise pulse rate maintained at approximately 120 beats per minute is considered a safe pulse. (Simply put, this is 20 beats in 10 sec or 12 beats in 6 sec.) As you begin the exercise program, keep your pulse rate around 100 to ensure that your body is reacting favorably to the new level of activity. As you progress in your program, you may adjust your exercise workout to increase your pulse to 132 (13 beats in 6 sec or 22 beats in 10 sec). As a general reference you may refer to Table 5.1 for the American Heart Association suggested target ranges. Remember, if you are taking one of the medications known as beta blockers, which affect your pulse rate, check with your physician for his or her suggestions.

It is important to be familiar with these guidelines for pulse rates, because as we grow older it is more and more dangerous to elevate our heart rate above the suggested maximum. Remember that the lower the resting heart rate the more efficiently the heart is working and the more exercise we can safely do. Even though it may seem strange, the best way to lower the heart rate is by elevating it for 15 to 20 min to its target heart rate through regular exercise, because this strengthens the heart muscle. A highly conditioned individual may have a heart rate as low as 50 beats per min, but for most of us the range is 70 to 75 beats per min. You need not be a mathematician to see that the well-conditioned heart is not working nearly so hard. During any period of aerobic activity, take your pulse periodically to make sure it is not elevated too high and to see that it is lowering and is approaching the resting heart rate at the end of the aerobic exercise session. If for some reason your pulse remains elevated for more than 2 hr, check with your doctor to see why. Again, always be aware of the warning signs of a heart attack (Table 5.2).

It is a good idea to tell your friends or family of your exercise plans; for example, the time of day you will exercise or the route you are walking. Also, carry some identification with you: your name and address and the phone number of a friend who can be contacted if you need help. Use the checklist that follows to remind yourself to make safety a part of your exercise plan.

- Have I allowed enough time (at least one hour) for my last meal to be digested?
- Did I drink water before and after exercising?
- Is my exercise attire suitable for the activity and the weather?
- Is my clothing brightly colored so that I am highly visible?
- Do I have identification with me?
- Have I informed a friend or neighbor of my exercise plans?
- Did I take my pulse at the beginning of the exercise period?
- Did I take my pulse at the halfway mark?
- Did I take my pulse at the end of my exercise session?

Safety tips that are more specific to the various activities will be found throughout the following chapters. If you make safety a regular part of your exercise program, you will avoid injury and increase your health benefits.

THE EXERCISE ROUTINE STEP-BY-STEP

Whatever exercise activity you choose, you should always adhere to the following sequence when you exercise.

1. Always begin your exercise session by walking for at least 5 min to start the process of "warming up the body."
2. Now do the 10- to 15-min basic warm-up routine (see Table 6.1). This will prepare all your joints and muscles for active exercise as well as strengthen and improve your balance and agility.
3. Follow with an activity that is continuous and rhythmic.

Monitor your workout to reach the desired target pulse rate or the rate of perceived exertion appropriate for you. Walking, cycling, dancing, and swimming are all excellent activities for this.

4. Cool down with the appropriate exercises (recommended in Table 6.2) and a short period of relaxation.

Correct Exercise Techniques

Some suggestions follow that will help you get the most benefit from your exercise program and will help you , as well, to avoid injuries or unnecessary soreness.

- *Do not bounce.* Use a smooth, slow movement when moving into an exercise and when moving from one exercise to another. Move into position and hold it. Do not bounce, because when you do you can cause tearing of the fibers in the muscle tissue. Do not force joints to the limits of their range of motion, and always remember to keep your movements smooth.
- *Do not lock.* Many of us have a tendency to lock our knees or elbows while standing and waiting, and sometimes even while exercising. Always protect your knees and elbows from hyperextension, that is, extreme or excessive straightening of a limb or body part. The joints in your knees and elbows are connected by means of ligaments and tendons, which have much less stretching capacity than muscles. In a young person, muscles can stretch 1 to 1½ times their resting length. The stretching capability of both the muscles and the ligaments and tendons decreases as we grow older. Thus, it is important not to force ligaments and tendons to stretch beyond their normal capacity.
- *Do not go too fast.* Exercises done at too fast a pace will not

build muscle strength, and doing exercises too rapidly may increase the possibility of injury.

- *Do exercises correctly.* Take time to learn to do the exercises the right way and then do them that way each time you work out. This is important because sometimes the beneficial effects of exercise are lessened when the exercise is done incorrectly. Sometimes the effects are even harmful. The following (Figs. 5.1 to 5.8) are exercises that should be avoided by the average person, together with acceptable alternatives for achieving the desired result. You will note that many of the "Don'ts" are old favorites of gym and drill instructors or have been traditionally included as part of the standard physical education classes. Nevertheless, research has shown that we should avoid them and stay with the proven alternatives to avoid injury.

Designing Your Individual Exercise Program

Now that all the information has been gathered, it is time to plan your individual program of exercise by working with the Exercise Program Worksheet in Table 5.4. (See also Appendix G.)

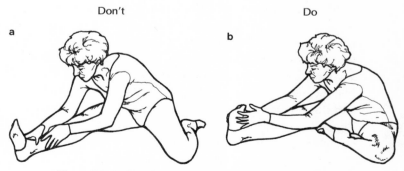

Figure 5.1. (a) Hurdler's stretch and (b) alternate leg stretch.

Don't   Do

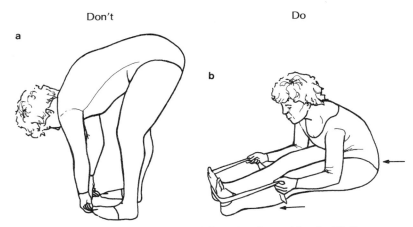

Figure 5.2. (a) Touching toes and (b) sitting forward bend with tie.

Don't   Do

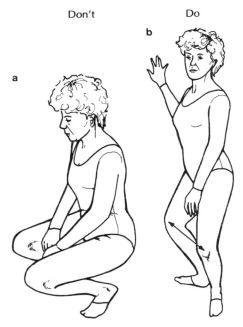

Figure 5.3. (a) Deep knee bends and (b) dancer's plié.

Don't   Do

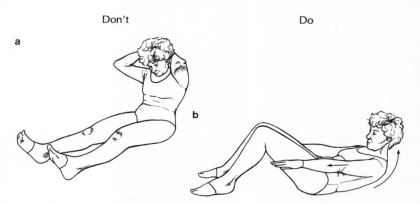

Figure 5.4. (a) Straight-leg sit-ups and (b) bent-knee sit-ups or curl-backs, curl-ups.

Don't   Do

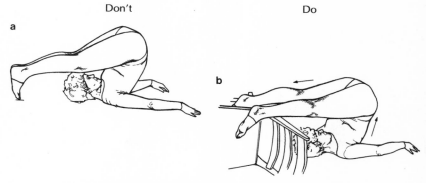

Figure 5.5. (a) Yoga plough and (b) rest legs on bench or wall.

Don't   Do

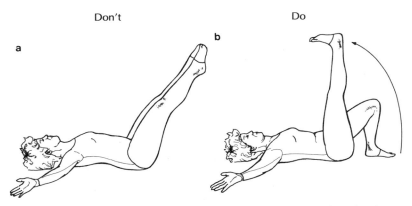

Figure 5.6. (a) Double leg lifts and (b) single leg lifts (opposite knee bent).

Don't   Do

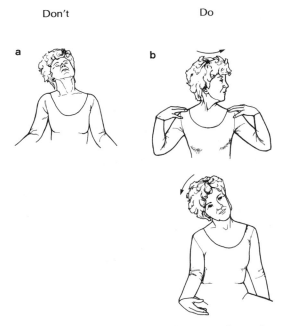

Figure 5.7. (a) Head rolls and (b) neck turns and stretches.

Don't   Do

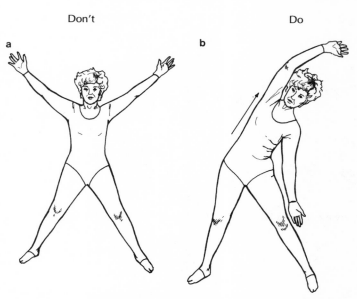

Figure 5.8. (a) Jumping jacks and (b) side leans with arms extended.

Look first at the AAHPERD Medical/Exercise Form from Chapter 2 (Fig. 2.1) for the information from your physician. Write down the comments and recommendations that were made. Also list what things you ought to be concerned about; e.g., high blood pressure, hernia. Now, write down the areas where you need to improve and the types of activities you want to do. Make a list of your personal goals. Do you need to lose or gain weight? Do you want to include a stress reduction activity like yoga or relaxation? What medications are you taking? Remember, if you have any questions about the effects of medications plus exercise on your body, consult your physician.

Now, looking at the five components of physical fitness previously discussed in Chapter 2 (flexibility, muscle strength and endurance, balance, cardiorespiratory endurance, and body composition), be sure you have included activities to help you improve in all areas. Also, take into consideration the four prescription factors described in Chapter 2. Be sure to plan your program to include a warm-up and cool-down period; do not give in to the temptation to skip these.

Now, refer to the results of your BSU self-appraisal tests. Is there information here to indicate an area of your body that needs special exercise? For example, lack of flexibility in the back, or lack of arm or abdominal strength? Plan your warm-up and cool-down exercises to exercise those areas that need it most.

Record Keeping

An important part of any activity program is recording the type of activity you do, the amount done, and your pulse rate at the beginning and end of the exercise session. Seeing your accomplishments down on paper is rewarding, and it helps keep you motivated to continue. Use the form (Table 5.5) presented here and also in Appendix J to record your exercise information. As you read further in this book about the various exercises or activities, there will be more discussion of how to record your progress.

SUMMARY

You are now well-informed and motivated to make exercise a part of your life. All that remains is for you to begin to exercise. The following chapters will help you discover the many ways in which you can enjoy being active. Whatever your interests, capabilities, or needs, there is something for you.

Table 5.4
Exercise Program Worksheet

1. Physician's comments and recommendations _____

   _____
   _____

2. I need to be concerned about _____

   _____

3. I enjoy doing _____
4. My personal goals are _____
5. The proper attire is _____
6. I need to _____ lose or _____ gain _____ pounds.
7. I will include a stress-reduction activity of _____
8. The medications I take may affect me during exercise.
   Yes _____ No _____. If yes, how will it affect me? _____

   _____

9. I need to improve flexibility in my (list body areas) _____ , _____

   _____ , _____ , _____

10. I need to improve muscle strength and endurance in my (list body areas) ____

    _____ , _____

11. I need to improve my balance. Yes _____ No _____
12. I plan to participate in _____ to improve my cardiorespiratory endurance.
13. My body composition needs improvement in the following ways _____
    14. To calculate the intensity level of my exercise workout:
        I. Resting pulse _____ + 20 beats = _____ .
        II. Estimate of maximal heart rate:

	220	220
	$-$Age	-55
Predicted maximal heart rate		165
Percent intensity	$\times$ %	(50%) $\times$ 0.5
Training or target heart rate		82.5

(continued)

Table 5.4. (*Continued*)

III. Karvonen equation		
Maximal heart rate	200	200
−Resting heart rate		−75
		125
× percent intensity (50%)		× 0.5
		62.5
+ resting heart rate		75.0
Training or target heart rate		137.5

    a. working at a 40% level my
       pulse rate will not exceed _____
    b. working at a 50% level my
       pulse rate will not exceed _____
    c. working at a 60% level my
       pulse rate will not exceed _____

15. My target heart rate is _____
16. I will begin my exercise program by working for _____ min _____ days a week.
17. My self-appraisal test results indicate I need to work on _____
_____
18. My warm-up exercises will last 5–10 min and I will do _____
_____
19. My cardiorespiratory segment will last 5 _____, 10 _____, 15 _____, or
20 _____ min and I will do _____
20. My cool-down exercise will last 5–20 min and I will do _____
_____

Table 5.5
Record of Progressive Conditioning Program

Date	Begin pulse[a]	Warm up	Pulse[a]	Mode[b]	Distance/time intensity	Exercise pulse[a]	Cool down

[a]Count pulse for 6 seconds, add a zero, and record.
[b]Write in: W, walking; SB, stationary bike; S, swimming; WJ, walk/jog; D, dance; J, jog; Y, yoga; TJ, Tai Ji; AQ, aquatic exercise.

BIBLIOGRAPHY

References

Borg, G., 1973, Perceived exertion: a note on history and methods, *Medicine and Science in Sports and Exercise* **5:**90–93.

Karvonen, M., Kentala, K., and Mustala, O., 1957, The effects of training on heart rate: a longitudinal study, *Annals of Medical and Experimental Biology* **35:** 307–315.

Kuntzelman, C. T., 1984, Exercise and sports in mid-life, in: Skalka, P., ed., *The American Medical Association Straight-Talk, No-Nonsense Guide to Health and Well-Being After 50*, New York, Random House.

Suggested Readings

Swan, P. D., and Spitler, D. L., 1989, Cardiac dimensions and physical profile of masters level swimmers, *Journal of Sports Medicine and Physical Fitness* **29**(1): 97–103.

CHAPTER 6

Building a Stronger
and More Flexible Body

For life is not to live, but to be well
Martial

This chapter will describe and illustrate exercises to strengthen
the muscles and improve the range of motion for the neck, shoulders, fingers, abdomen, back, legs, and feet. Please remember the
basic guidelines discussed in Chapter 4, because these exercise
guidelines apply now as well. Some of these exercises are from
sports, hatha yoga, and dance. Each exercise presented will have a
number, the written description, a drawing, the number of repetitions for doing the exercises for both the beginner level and the
challenge level, a breathing pattern, and sometimes specific precautions. If you are beginning an exercise program after not
having exercised for awhile, we recommend that you start at the
beginner's level. If you have been exercising regularly, we suggest
that you try the challenge level; if you are comfortable doing the

exercises without any pain or distress, that level will probably be all right for you. Many of the exercises can be done either while standing or sitting. If you choose to do the exercises while sitting, use a firm, armless chair with a straight back that will allow you to sit with your feet firmly on the floor.

The Basic 40 exercises form the core of the Basic Warm-up Program and The Basic Cool-down Program. These exercises will be referred to throughout the rest of the book by the number. Whenever you have a question about how to do an exercise please refer to this section. The Basic Warm-up exercises will be identified by a W and the Basic Cool-down exercises by a C.

NECK

1. **Head Turns** (Fig. 6.1)   W
    1. Stand or sit with back erect and fingertips resting on shoulders
    2. Slowly turn head only from side to side. The rest of the body remains still.
       Breath pattern: Inhale through the nose as you turn to the

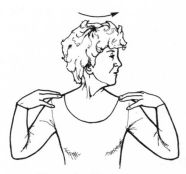

Figure 6.1. Head turn.

side and exhale through the mouth as you bring the
head back to center.

Level

Beginner: Do 5 to each side, adding 1 per week.

Challenge: Do 10 to each side.

2. **Head Tilts** (Fig. 6.2)   W

   1. Stand or sit with back erect
   2. Tilt head to each side for 2–4 counts and then lift back to
      center.

      Breath pattern: Inhale through the nose as you tilt to the side
         and exhale through the mouth as you bring the head
         back to center.

   Level

   Beginner: Do 5 to each side, adding 1 per week

   Challenge: Do 10 to each side.

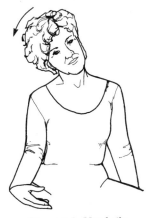

Figure 6.2. Head tilt.

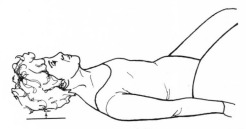

Figure 6.3. Head lift.

3. **Head Lift** (Fig. 6.3)
    1. Lie on the back with knees bent.
    2. Lift the head 1–2 in from the floor and hold.
    3. Do not tilt the chin toward the chest.
       Breath pattern: Inhale when lifting the head and exhale
          while counting.
       Level
          Beginner: Hold while counting to 4 out loud.
          Challenge: Hold while counting to 8 out loud.

4. **Head Lift and Turn** (Fig. 6.4)
    1. Lying on back with knees bent, lift head 1–2 inches from the
       floor, holding.
    2. Turn the head to the side, and back to the center.
    3. Then turn the head to the other side, and then back to the
       center and lower to the floor.

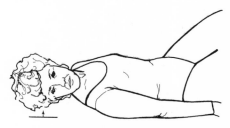

Figure 6.4. Head lift and turn.

Breath pattern: Inhale through the nose as you lift head, and exhale through the mouth as you hold and count. Inhale as you turn to the side and exhale as you turn back to the center.

Level

Beginner: Lift and hold for 2 counts, turn to each side for 2 counts.

Challenge: Increase the count by 1 while you are holding the head off the floor in the center position and in the two turning positions.

SHOULDERS

5. **Single Arm Swings** (Fig. 6.5)   W

   1. Stand or sit on an armless chair, keep back erect.
   2. Swing the arms forward and backward gently.

   Breath pattern: Inhale as the arms come forward and exhale as the arms swing back.

   Level

   Beginner: Do 5 with each arm.

   Challenge: Do 10 with each arm.

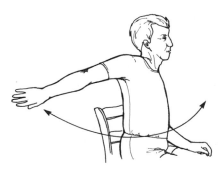

Figure 6.5. Arm swing.

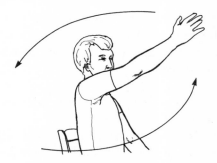

Figure 6.6. Arm circles.

6. **Arm Circles** (Fig. 6.6)   W
   1. Arms can circle both forward and back.
   2. When standing, allow the knees to bend and the body to
      flow with the movement.
   3. Arms can also circle in opposition at the same time the right
      arm comes forward, the left arm circles to the back.
      Breath pattern: Inhale as arm swings forward and exhale as
         arm swings back.
      Level
         Beginner: 5 swings with each arm.
         Challenge: 10 swings with each arm.

7. **Wall Walk and Slide** (Fig. 6.7)   C
   1. Facing the wall with elbows straight, walk your fingers up
      the wall as far as you can comfortably reach. (Fig. 6.7a).
   2. Slowly back away, "dragging" your arms and hands down

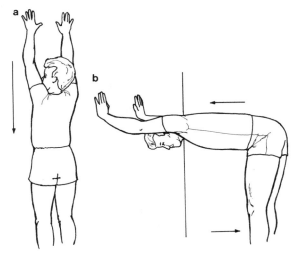

Figure 6.7. (a) Wall walk and (b) slide.

the wall until you have your back horizontal and palms on the wall with arms straight (Fig. 6.7b). Practice Step "2" with your hands holding on to a chair back, a table top, or a counter.

3. Hold the position and enjoy the opening of the shoulder girdle.
4. Round the back and push back from the wall to a standing position.

Breath pattern: Breathe deeply and relax into the stretches as you exhale allowing the body to let go.

Level

Beginner: Do 2 times.

Challenge: Do 4 times.

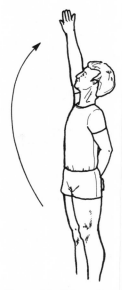

Figure 6.8. Side wall walk.

8. **Side Wall Walk** (Fig. 6.8)
   1. Stand with your side to the wall and "walk" your arm up as far as it will go.
   2. Look to see where your hand was and watch for improvement as your hand is eventually able to walk further.
   3. Repeat on the other side with the other arm.
      Breath pattern: Breathe deeply as you do the "walking" up the wall.
      Level
        Beginner: Do 2–4 times.
        Challenge: Do 6 times.

9. **Shoulder Shrugs** (Fig. 6.9)   C
   1. Standing or sitting with the back erect, first lift the shoulders up.

2. Now lift the shoulders back as far as they will comfortably go.
   Breath pattern: Inhale as you lift and exhale as you lower the
     shoulders.
   Level:
     Beginner: Do 2–4 times
     Challenge: Do 6 times.
10. **Behind the Back Tie Stretch** (Fig. 6.10)   C
    1. Holding a tie in your right hand, extend the right hand and
       arm upward so the elbow and the upper arm are near the
       head.
    2. Bend the elbow, dropping the tie down the back.
    3. With the left arm behind the back, grasp the tie with the left
       hand and gently pull up with the right hand and down
       with the left in a gentle up and down motion.
    4. Release and repeat on the other side.
       Breath pattern: Breathe deeply throughout the movements.
       Level:
         Beginner: Do the up and down stretch 2 times with each
         arm.
         Challenge: Do the up and down stretch 3–4 times with
         both arms.

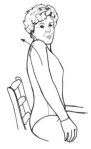

Figure 6.9. Shoulder shrugs.

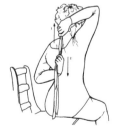

Figure 6.10. Tie stretch.

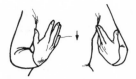

Figure 6.11. Hand shaking.

HANDS

11. **Shaking** (Fig. 6.11)
    With hands relaxed, gently shake them.

12. **Finger Circles** (Fig. 6.12)
    1. With fingers curved and the fingertips of each hand touching.
    2. Separate each pair of fingers an inch and then have this pair of fingers circle each other 4–5 times and then reverse the circling direction and touch them back together.
    3. Repeat on the next pair of fingers.
    4. While one pair is circling each other, the other 4 pairs are maintaining contact.
       Breath pattern: Breathe normally throughout.

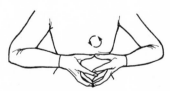

Figure 6.12. Finger circles.

PECTORAL MUSCLES OF THE CHEST

13. **Chest Stretch in Doorway** (Fig. 6.13)   C
    1. Place hand against a wall or doorway with the arm raised
       and straight.
    2. Keep shoulders down and slowly turn your torso away
       from the wall.
    3. Repeat with the other arm.
       Breath pattern: Breathe deeply and normally as you hold in
           the stretch position.
       Level
         Beginner: Do 2 each side.
         Challenge: Do 4 each side.

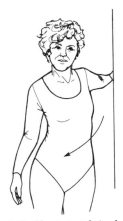

Figure 6.13. Chest stretch in doorway.

14. **Wall Push-up** (Fig. 6.14)   W
    1. Facing the wall place palms at shoulder height and hold the body firm. Feet are placed a comfortable distance back from the wall. (Do NOT do in stockings as your feet will slip.)
    2. Bend the elbows and bring the body toward the wall.
       Breath pattern: Do not hold the breath. Inhale on Step 1 and count out loud as you exhale on Step 2.
       Level
         Beginner: Do 5 times
         Challenge: Do 10 times.

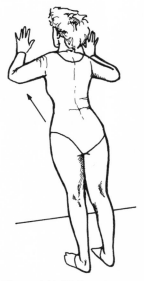

Figure 6.14. Wall push-up.

15. **Forearm Press Isometrically** (Fig. 6.15)
    1. Press arms together from fingertips to elbows.
    2. As you press, lift elbows up toward the chin.
    3. Lower and relax
       Breath pattern: Inhale as arms move into the position and
          exhale as you press. Inhale as arms are lowered and
          relaxed and exhale as you repeat the press and lift. Do
          not hold your breath.
       Level
          Beginner: Do 4 times
          Challenge: Do 6 times.

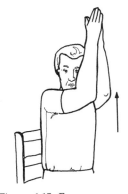

Figure 6.15. Forearm press.

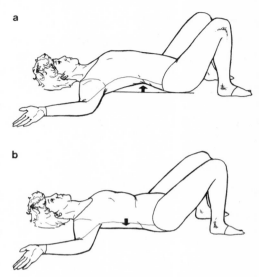

Figure 6.16. Pelvic tilt. (a) Starting position and (b) doing the tilt.

BACK

16. **Pelvic Tilt** (Fig. 6.16)   W
    1. Lie on back, knees bent, feet flat on the floor (Fig. 6.16a)
    2. Contract the abdominal muscles and press the lumbar area
       of the spine to the floor and hold for 5 counts (Fig. 6.16b).
       Breath pattern: Inhale and contract and as you exhale and
          tilt you count out loud to five. Then inhale as you relax
          between repeats and always exhale as you tilt and count
          out loud while holding the contraction.
       Level
          Beginner: Do 5 tilts.
          Challenge: Do 8–10 tilts.

17. **Knees to Chest** (Fig. 6.17)   C
    A. Single knee to chest
    1. Lie on back, with knees bent.
    2. Bring one bent leg toward the chest.

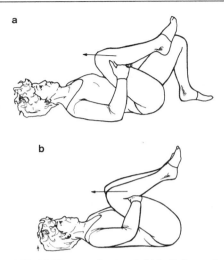

Figure 6.17. (a) Knee to chest and (b) both knees to chest.

3. Clasp hands behind the knee and gently press leg closer to the chest.
4. Hold for 5 counts and repeat with the other leg.
   Breath pattern: Inhale as you bring leg up. Exhale and count out loud to five as you press to chest. Inhale as you change to other leg. Exhale as you press and count out loud to five. Do recommended number of repeats in this way.
   Level
      Beginner: Do 4 with each leg.
      Challenge: Do 8 with each leg.
B. Both knees to chest
1. Lie on back with knees bent.
2. Bring both knees to the chest with the hands behind knees.
3. Gently pull legs toward chest, lift head, and hold while you count out loud to 5.
   Breath pattern: Same as above.
   Level
      Beginner: Do 4 times.
      Challenge: Do 8 times.

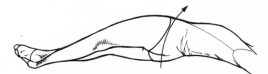

Figure 6.18. Crocodile twist.

18. **Crocodile Twist** (Fig. 6.18)   C
    1. Lying on back with legs straight, cross the right ankle over
       the left and keep arms straight out from shoulders with
       palms up.
    2. Now gently twist legs to the right and turn the head to the
       left.
    3. Hips will lift from the floor a bit, but keep the shoulders
       down because this produces a gentle stretch.
    4. Repeat with the left ankle on top of the right.
       Breath pattern: Inhale as you twist over to the side and
          exhale as you return to the center starting position.
       Level
          Beginner: Do 4 twists to each side.
          Challenge: Do 6 twists to each side.

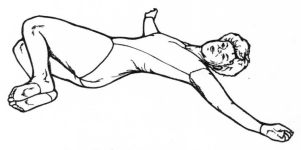

Figure 6.19. Knee-overs.

19. **Knee-overs** (Fig. 6.19)   W and C
    1. Lying on back with knees bent and feet flat on the floor.
    2. Lower both legs down to the right and turn the head to the left.
    3. Then lift back to starting position.
    4. Repeat taking the bent knees over to the left.
       Breath pattern: Inhale as you lower knees to the side. Exhale as you lift them back to center position.

20. **Back push-up** (Fig. 6.20)   W
    1. Lying on back with knees bent and feet flat on floor near the buttocks, palms on floor by bent legs.
    2. Contract muscles of abdomen, buttocks, thighs, and internal muscles as you inhale.
    3. Slowly lift the back and arms up from the floor until arms are resting on the floor above the head and back is as high as you can lift.
    4. Exhale as you lower back to floor one vertebra at a time and the arms lower also until you are in the starting position.
       Count to four as you go up and to four as you lower.
       Breath pattern: Inhale as you lift up and exhale as you lower.
       Level
         Beginner: Do 4 times.
         Challenge: Do 6–8 times.

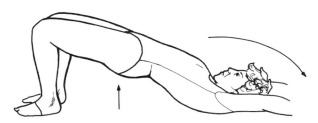

Figure 6.20. Back push-up.

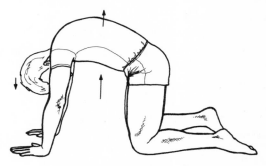

Figure 6.21. Cat.

21. **Cat** (Fig. 6.21)   W
    1. Kneel with the palms of the hands directly under the shoulders and knees directly under the hips.
    2. Contract the abdominal muscles and let the back arch up toward the ceiling as you lower your head.
    3. Lower the back and stretch the head forward.
       (Hint: If you have problems with your wrists and placing your palms flat on the floor is uncomfortable, make a fist and try it that way.)
       Breath pattern: Inhale as the back lowers and the head comes forward. Exhale as the abdominal muscles contract and the back arches up.
       Level
       Beginner: Do 4 times.
       Challenge: Do 6–8 times.

22. **Pose of the Child** (Fig. 6.22)   W
    1. Kneeling and resting the abdomen and chest on the thighs.
    2. Keep the hips by your heels if possible and lower the forehead toward the floor.
    3. Use a pillow under your head if you want. Let the arms rest beside the lower legs.
    4. Stay in the pose as long as you are comfortable.
    5. Come up very slowly.

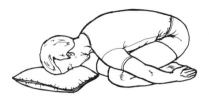

Figure 6.22. Pose of a child.

Breath pattern: Inhale, then as you exhale allow the back to relax and gently stretch. Breathe fully and deep.
Level
All just enjoy the pose while you are comfortable in it.

ABDOMEN

23. **Standing Cat Stretch** (Fig. 6.23)
    1. Stand with feet hip-width apart, hands on relaxed knees.
    2. Sink the lower back into an arch.
    3. Contract abdominals up and drop head forward.
       Breath pattern: Inhale as the back is lowered, exhale as back is lifted.

    Level
       Beginner: Do 4 times.
       Challenge: Do 6–8 times.

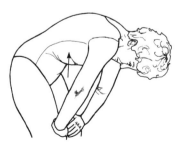

Figure 6.23. Standing cat.

24. **Sit-backs** (Fig. 6.24)   W
    1. Sit on floor with knees bent, hands resting on knees, and feet flat on floor. (Also, you can place a towel on top of feet and put them under a sofa.)
    2. Remember not to hold your breath
    3. Contract abdominals and lower the back until you are at a 45° angle. Hold while counting out loud to four (Fig. 6.24a).
    4. Lower the back until you are on the sacrum (Fig. 6.24b). Round the back and count out loud to 4 as you hold.
    5. Lower further until the shoulders are only 1 in to ½ in off the floor (Fig. 6.24c). Count out loud to four.
    6. Lower the back to the floor, straighten legs, stretch arms over head, take a deep breath, and stretch entire body.
    7. Turn over on side and sit up.
       Breath pattern: Breathe continuously during the exercise.
       Level
          Beginner: Do 4 times and add 1 per day until doing 8.

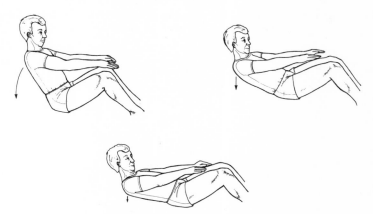

Figure 6.24. Sit-backs.

Challenge: When the sitting-back phase becomes easy, reverse the procedure and come up into a sitting position. Remember to bend the knees and contract the abdominal muscles.

25. **Elbows to Knees** (Fig. 6.25)
    Caution: Go slow if you have sore neck muscles.
    1. Lie on your back with knees bent, hands supporting your head, and feet resting on a stool or chair.
    2. Try to reach knees with elbows on a slow count of eight (Fig.6.25a).
    3. Do 4 times.
    4. Then touch opposite elbow to opposite knee (Fig. 6.25b).
    5. Do 4 times, exhaling when elbow touches or moves toward knee.
    6. Stretch out arms and legs and breathe deeply.
       Breath pattern: Inhale when lying on back. Exhale when elbows move toward knees.
       Level
       Beginner: Do a total of 8 times.
       Challenge: Hold legs in the air, with knees bent and ankles crossed. Do the exercise in this position. Repeat 6–8 times each movement.

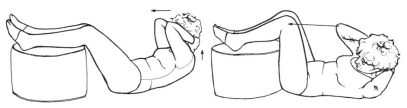

Figure 6.25. Elbows toward knees.

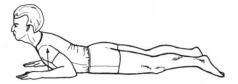

Figure 6.26. Cool-down stretching.

26. **Cool-down Stretch** (Fig. 6.26)   W
Caution: If you have back problems go very slowly and not
very high.
Hint: Keep abdominal muscles contracted and do not let the
back sag.
1. Lie face down on floor, palms under shoulders, legs
   straight.
2. Gently lift chest up from floor as you inhale.
3. Keep pelvis on the floor, exhale, and lower.
4. Do 1 time and if you feel comfortable do 2–3 more.

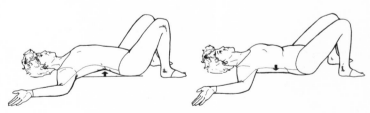

Figure 6.27. Pelvic tilt.

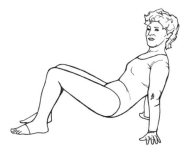

Figure 6.28. Buttock firmer.

BUTTOCKS

27. **Pelvic Tilt** (Fig. 6.27)

    For directions refer to Exercise 16.

28. **Buttock Firmer** (Fig. 6.28)

    1. Sit on floor with back erect, arms braced slightly behind, and fingers pointing away from the body. Knees are bent and apart and feet are flat on the floor.
    2. Contract buttocks and tuck pelvis under.
    3. Lift 6 in off the floor, lower, and then repeat.

       Breath pattern: Inhale in starting position and exhale up to lift. Inhale as you lower down and exhale as you raise up on the repeats.

       Level

       Beginner: Do 6 times, rest, and do 4 more.

       Challenge: Do the same as for Beginner level, but lift pelvis higher until the thighs are almost parallel to the floor. Do 6 times, rest and do 4 more.

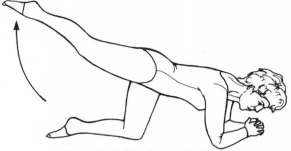

Figure 6.29. Kneeling single lift.

29. **Kneeling Single Leg Lifts** (Fig. 6.29).
    Hint: Keep abdominal muscles contracted and do not let the back sag.
    1. Begin on your knees and forearms.
    2. Straighten right leg and lift upward, and then lower.
    3. Repeat with the left leg.
       Level
           Beginner: Do 8 to 10 times with each leg.
               Breath pattern: Inhale, then lift the leg as you exhale, lower leg and inhale.
           Challenge: Assume same position as for Beginner level. Now, with the leg extended, hold it there and then bend the knee, bringing the heel toward the buttock. Do 8 to 10 times with each leg.
               Breath pattern: Inhale as you lift the leg, exhale as you bend the knee, and inhale as you straighten the leg.

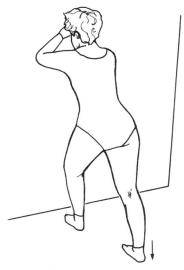

Figure 6.30. Lower leg stretch at wall.

LEGS

30. **Lower Leg Stretch at Wall** (Fig. 6.30)   C
    1. Stand facing the wall with the forearms resting on the wall and feet in a stride position (left foot forward and left knee bent and the right foot back). Point the toes of both feet to wall.
    2. Have the heel of the back leg (the right one) touching the floor so that your leg stretches gently.
    3. Change so that the left foot is back and the right is forward. Breath pattern: Breathe normally and relax into the stretch. Level
        Beginner: Do 3 each leg.
        Challenge: Do 6 each leg.

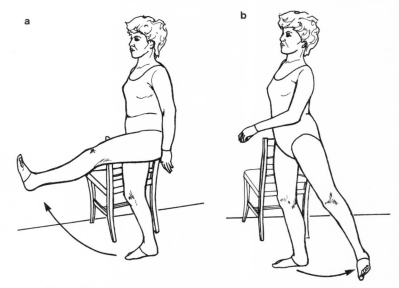

Figure 6.31. (a) Standing leg swings and (b) standing leg circles.

31. **Standing Leg Swings and Circles** (Fig. 6.31)   W
    1. Stand with your side to a wall, chair, or table and place hand there for stability.
    2. Swing the outside leg forward and back, keeping the trunk erect.
    3. Circle the leg forward and then backward.
    4. Repeat with the other leg.
       Breath pattern: Keep breath flowing smoothly throughout the movement.
       Level
          Beginner: Do 8 swings and 8 circles forward and 8 swings and 8 circles back.
          Challenge: Increase the height of the swings and the size of the circles.

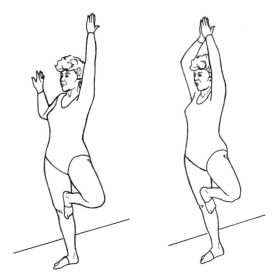

Figure 6.32. Tree balance.

32. **Tree Balance** (Fig. 6.32)   W
    1. Stand with your side to a wall, table, or chair and hand placed there for stability.
    2. Place the sole of the foot of the outside leg against the thigh or knee of the supporting leg.
    3. Keep trunk erect and head up.
    4. Hold balance position for a count of ten.
    5. Repeat with other leg.
       Breath pattern: Keep breath flowing smoothly during balancing.
       Level
          Beginner: Do 2 times with each leg.
          Challenge: Hold the pose for a count of 20; also can remove the hand from the wall, table, or chair and extend both arms up over your head.

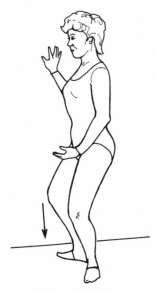

Figure 6.33. Plié.

33. **Plié** (Fig. 6.33)
   1. Stand with your side to a chair or table with hand lightly resting for stability.
   2. Bend the knees slightly, keeping the center of the knee in line with the middle of each foot.
   3. As you raise up contract the muscles of your quadriceps to lift you, feeling as if you are squeezing the legs together. Breath pattern: Inhale as you lower and exhale as you raise back to the starting position.
   Level
   Beginner: Do 8 times
   Challenge: Do 12 times.

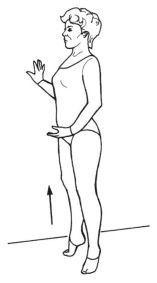

Figure 6.34. Relevé.

34. **Relevé** (Fig. 6.34)
    1. Stand by a chair or table with hands resting lightly for stability.
    2. Raise onto the balls of the feet, lifting the heels off the floor and spreading your weight over all ten toes.
    3. Lower slowly and smoothly (do not flex the knees).
       Breath pattern: Inhale as you raise up and exhale as you lower back to starting position.
       Level
       Beginner: Do 8 times.
       Challenge: Do 12 times.

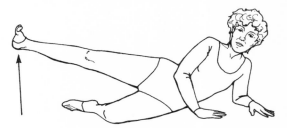

Figure 6.35. Side leg lift.

35. **Side Leg Lifts** (Fig. 6.35)   W
    1. Lie on the side with the bottom leg bent at the knee and the
       arms supporting the body.
    2. Lift the top leg until it is at the height of the shoulders, then
       lower.
       Breath pattern: Inhale as you lift the leg and exhale as you
           lower.
       Level
           Beginner: Do 8 times with each leg.
           Challenge: Alternate pointing toes and flexing feet. Do 8
               times with each leg.

36. **Inner Thigh Firmer** (Fig. 6.36)   W
    1. Lie on the side and place the bent top leg so the foot is on
       floor in back of knee of straight bottom leg.
    2. Hold ankle in top hand while supporting the body on the
       elbow of the bottom arm.
    3. Flex feet and lift bottom leg (Fig. 6.36a).
    4. Repeat on the other side lifting other leg.
       Breath pattern: Inhale as you lift the leg and exhale as you
           lower.

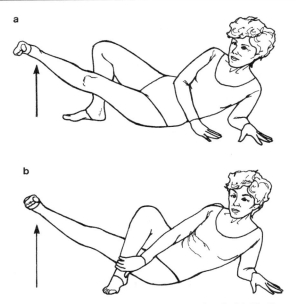

Figure 6.36. Inner thigh firmer. (a) Beginner level. (b) Challenge level.

Level

Beginner: Do 10 times each leg.

Challenge: Do 10 times with top bent leg placed with the foot in front of the straight bottom leg (Fig. 6.36b). Repeat 10 times with other leg.

FEET AND ANKLES

Hint: It is best to do these barefoot.

Breath pattern: Breathe normally throughout all the following exercises.

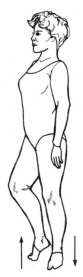

Figure 6.37. Prancing.

37. **Prancing** (Fig. 6.37)   W
     1. Standing erect, raise up on to the ball and toes of one foot
        as the other foot remains flat on the floor.
     2. Slowly transfer the weight through the arch as you change
        from one foot to the other.
        Level
           Beginner: Do 10 prances with each foot.
           Challenge: Do 20 prances with each foot.

38. **Ankle Circles—Standing** (Fig. 6.38)
     1. Stand with the weight on the right foot and let the toes of
        the left foot remain on the floor.
     2. Slowly circle the leg, allowing the ankle to rotate and
        stretch. Reverse the direction
     3. Repeat on the other foot.

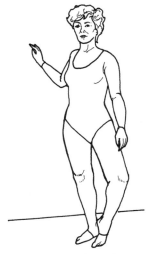

Figure 6.38. Ankle circles, standing.

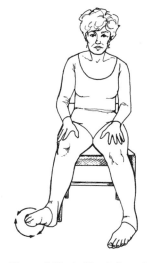

Figure 6.39. Ankle circles, sitting.

Level

Beginner: Do 5 circles in each direction with each foot.

Challenge: Do 10 circles in each direction with each foot.

39. **Ankle Circles—Sitting** (Fig. 6.39)

1. With legs still, rotate the feet in circles, moving at the ankle joint.
2. Reverse the direction.
3. Repeat circles in each direction.

   Level

   Beginner: Do a total of 10 with each foot in both directions.

   Challenge: Do a total of 20 with each foot in both directions.

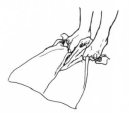

Figure 6.40. Towel scrunch.

40. **Towel Scrunch** (Fig. 6.40)
    1. Sitting or standing with a towel under the toes.
    2. Grab the towel with your toes and pull the end of it toward you.
    3. Straighten out the towel and repeat.
       Level
          Beginner: Do 4 times.
          Challenge: Do 8 times.

WARM-UP AND COOL-DOWN EXERCISE PROGRAMS

Now you can refer to the following tables (Tables 6.1 and 6.2) for a listing of the exercises recommended for a thorough warm up and cool down. It is important not to rush or neglect these two phases of your exercise program. In the tables the exercise is identified by name, number (which also refers to the figure), and page number if you want the complete instructions or if you want to refresh your memory. Beg. refers to the beginner level and chal. refers to the challenge level, with the number referring to the repetitions of each exercise recommended.

Table 6.1
Basic Warm-up Program

1. Begin walking to music around the room for 2–5 min.

2. While walking, sitting in a chair, or standing do:
   a. Head Turns, #1; beg.: 5, chal.: 10 (p. 100)
   b. Head Tilts, #2; beg.: 5, chal.: 10 (p. 101)
   c. Single Arm Swings, #5; beg.: 5, chal.: 10 (p. 103)
   d. Arm Circles, #6; Forward and back, beg.: 5, chal.: 10 (p. 106)

3. Standing by a wall or chair do:
   a. Standing Leg Swings and Circles, #31; beg.: 8 of each, chal.: 10 each but increase height of swing and size of circle (p. 124)
   b. Prancing, #37; beg. and chal.: 10 (p. 130)
   c. Tree Balance, #32; beg.: 2–4, chal.: Hold while counting to 20 and repeat (p. 125)
   d. Wall Push-ups, #14; beg.: 5, chal.: 10 (p. 110)

4. On mats or padded floor do:
   a. Side Leg Lifts, #35; beg.: 8, chal.: 8 and alternate pointing toes and flexing (bringing toes toward leg) the foot of the leg being lifted (p. 128)
   b. Inner Thigh Firmer, #36; beg.: 10, chal.: 10 and place the foot of the bent leg in front of the bottom leg (p. 128)

5. Lying on the back on mats or padded floor do:
   a. Pelvic Tilt, #16; beg.: 5, chal.: 10 (p. 112)
   b. Knee-overs, #19; beg.: 4, chal.: 8 (p. 115)
   c. Back Push-up, #20; beg.: 4, chal.: 8 (p. 115)
   d. Roll to side and come up to sitting position slowly.

6. Sitting on mats or padded floor do:
   a. Sit-backs, #24; beg.: 4 (When four becomes easy add one until you gradually are doing eight.), chal.: when doing 8 at the beginner level is easy, come up from the down position reversing the procedure (p. 118)

7. Lying on abdomen on mat or padded floor do:
   a. Cool-down Stretch, #26; beg.: 1, chal.: 3 (p. 120)

8. Kneeling on mat or padded floor do:
   a. Cat, #21; beg.: 4, chal.: 8 (p. 116)

9. Lying on back on mat or padded floor do:
   a. Knees to Chest, #17A; beg.: 5, chal.: 10 (p. 112)

Table 6.2
Basic Cool-down Program

1. Walk at a slower pace, or if riding on an exercise bike, ride at a slower pace. Standing, do:

2. Single Arm Swings, #5; beg.: 5, chal.: 10 (p. 103)

3. Wall Walk and Slide, #7; beg.: 2–4, chal.: 6 (p. 104)

4. Shoulder Shrugs, #9; beg.: 2–4, chal.: 6 (p. 106)

5. Chest Stretch in Doorway, #13; beg.: 3 each side, chal.: 6 each side (p. 109)

6. Lower Leg Stretch at Wall, #30; beg.: 3 each leg, chal.: 6 each leg (p. 123)

Lying on padded floor or mat, do:

7. Knees to Chest, #17; beg.: 5, chal.: 8 (p. 112)

8. Crocodile Twist, # 18; beg.: 4, chal.: 8 (p. 114)

9. Knee-overs, #19; beg.: 4 to each side, chal.: 8 to each side (p. 115)

10. Pose of the Child, #22; Both beg. and chal. stay as long as comfortable (p. 116)

Now your entire body has been gently stretched and strengthened and is ready for the next step—the conditioning workout of your choice.

Following your conditioning or aerobic workout you should do the all purpose cool-down stretches or the ones recommended for that specific activity.

SUMMARY

Now that you have become familiar with the Basic 40 exercises for strength and flexibility, you will want to move on to the next chapter for a very different approach to achieving a healthy mind and body.

BIBLIOGRAPHY

Suggested Readings

Corbin, D., and Metal-Corbin, J., 1990, *Reach For It*, 2nd ed., Dubuque, Iowa, Eddie Bowers, Publishing, Inc.

Rikkers, R., 1986, *Seniors on the Move*, Champaign, Illinois, Human Kinetics Publishers, Inc.

Chapter 7

Soft and Gentle

Gentle in method
Resolute in action
from the Latin

This chapter will present a softer approach to exercise via activities that come from around the world. Included are Hatha Yoga from India, Tai Ji Chuan from China, and the Feldenkrais Awareness through Movement System, which was developed by a Russian who emigrated to Israel.

Relaxation, stress-reduction techniques, pain control, and imagery will also be discussed. All of these activities can improve the breathing, habits, concentration, posture, balance, flexibility,

137

and muscle tone of those participating. Each of these approaches to body awareness will be discussed separately.

HATHA YOGA

Hatha Yoga developed more than 5,000 years ago in India and is made up of *asanas*, which are static, slow, stretching exercises; *pranayama*, which is the breathing technique; and *relaxation*. When beginning a program of Hatha Yoga, the following guidelines are suggested so that maximum benefits may be achieved.

Basic Guidelines

1. It is best to be in loose-fitting clothes (no girdles).
2. It is best to be bare foot so that your sensory awareness and balance are enhanced.
3. Many of the exercises or poses can be done while sitting in a chair.
4. The standing poses all can be done beside a chair for additional support if desired.
5. The breath is always coordinated with the exercise being done; inhaling through the nose on expanding movements and exhaling on contracting movements. The breath is not held.
6. It is important to concentrate on how the body is responding to the exercise; how it feels. Ask yourself questions such as, "Am I more flexible today?" or "Do I have less tension in my back?"
7. The *asanas* done on the floor should be done on a padded

surface such as an exercise mat or carpet to protect the back and hips.

Hatha Yoga is an appropriate activity for all. It should be done in a slow and gentle manner. It is noncompetitive, does not require expensive equipment, and can be done anywhere—on the beach or at the grandchildren's home. Several of the Hatha Yoga poses have been described in Chapter 6 and are part of the basic warm-up and cool-down routines. When those poses are mentioned in these yoga routines the figure number is listed together with the page number so that you may refer to them for further instructions. Now, we invite you to enjoy a typical Hatha Yoga class by doing the following lesson. The traditional poses have occasionally been modified to better meet your exercise needs.

Hatha Yoga Routine

Sitting on a firm chair with a straight back do:
Deep Breathing
Benefits: The whole body, and the respiratory system in particular, benefits from the deep breathing.

Precautions: Do not hyperventilate or hold the breath.

Directions
1. Sit quietly, with the hands, arms, and shoulders relaxed, eyes lightly closed, and both feet flat on the floor.
2. Inhale through the nose allowing the abdomen to expand and the lungs to fill as completely as they can.
3. Slowly exhale through the mouth or the nose if you desire.

Head Turns and Head Tilts (Figs. 6.1 and 6.2, pp. 100, 101)
Benefits: Improve the range of motion in the neck.

Precautions: Go very slowly if you have any problems with the cervical vertebrae. Do not force.

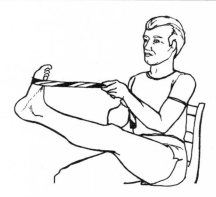

Figure 7.1. Leg tie stretch.

Leg Tie Stretch (Fig. 7.1)
   Benefits: Improves flexibility of the knees, ankles, and hips.
   Precautions: Avoid this exercise if you have had a hip re-
   placement.
   Directions
   1. Bend the knee and place a necktie under the ball of the foot
      (not the arch), holding the ends of the tie in your hands.
   2. Straighten the leg and slowly raise the leg until a gentle
      stretch is felt. Hold and breathe normally. Lower slowly.
   3. Repeat with the other leg.

Now do the following while standing:
   Postural Alignment (Fig. 7.2)
   Suggestion: Do this in front of a mirror, if possible. This
      alignment is the basis for all the standing poses.
   Benefits: Improves posture and strengthens feet.
   Precautions: Don't lock the knees or leave the arms raised for
      too long.
   Directions
   1. Stand erect in bare feet with both feet facing straight ahead
      and under the hips.

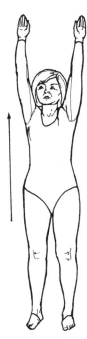

Figure 7.2. Postural alignment.

2. Tighten the quadriceps muscles of the thigh (front). Contract the abdominals, tuck the pelvis slightly under, and lift the chest.
3. Keep the head level and over the spine—not forward. Shoulders are down and back.
4. Slowly raise the arms so they are pointing to the ceiling. The fingers are straight but are not held rigid. Also, do NOT hunch the shoulders—keep them down from the ears.
5. Notice a lengthening of the spine and the rib cage lifting.
6. Breathe deeply and lower the arms slowly.

Tree (Fig. 6.32, p. 125)

> **Benefits**: Strengthens legs and feet and improves balance and posture.
>
> **Precautions**: If you have inner ear or other balance problems that may be induced by medication, hold on to a chair back, table, counter, or wall.

Abdominal Lift (Fig. 7.3)

Do this pose 2–3 times daily upon arising.

> **Benefits**: Tones abdominal muscles, gently massages the internal organs, and aids in digestion and relief of constipation.
>
> **Precautions**: Do not do if you have an ulcer, hernia, or high blood pressure. No one should do this pose on a full stomach.

Directions

1. Stand with the legs apart, knees bent, and hands resting just above the knees.
2. The abdominal muscles are going to contract, pulling inward toward the spine. To help this happen exhale through the mouth saying "HA" and *then* contract and hold while counting to three. Release the contraction and take a deep breath.
3. Repeat two more times.

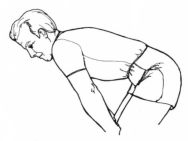

Figure 7.3. Abdominal lift.

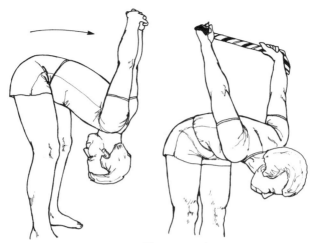

Figure 7.4. Chest expansion.

Chest Expansion (Fig. 7.4)

   Benefits: Improves flexibility of the shoulders, elbows, wrists, and spine and brings blood to the head, which can be invigorating.

   Precautions: Do not do if you have glaucoma, retina problems, or recent eye surgery. Do not do if you have problems with dizziness. If you have high or low blood pressure do not stay in the pose very long.

   Directions

   1. You can use a necktie to assist you or you can join your hands if this does not strain the joints of your wrist, elbow, and hands.

   2. To begin, stand erect and with your arms at shoulder height; bring them out to the side and then behind you, grabbing hold of the tie or your other hand.

   3. Straighten your arms slowly if you can do so comfortably and inhale.

4. Now bend forward slowly as you EXHALE, letting the arms rise toward the ceiling and breathing NORMALLY.
5. Do not lock the knees.
6. Come up slowly.

Variation (Fig. 7.4b):

1. If you are comfortable in the position you can add a small, slow circle of the head. This helps the muscles of the neck to stretch gently. You are using the weight of the head as it is hanging down to add to the lengthening of the neck.

Small Cobra (Fig. 6.26, p. 120, Cool-down Stretch)
Do 2–3 times
   Benefits: Improves flexibility of the spine, shoulders, and neck and strengthens the arms
   Precautions: If you have problems with your lower back do not force yourself to lift very high.
   Directions
   1. Lie on abdomen with chin on the mat and palms under the shoulders.
   2. Contract the muscles around the navel and INHALE as you lift the chest up slightly from the mat.
   3. Keep the shoulders down from the ears and gaze forward and up slightly. Keep the pelvis on the floor.
   4. Lower slowly and with control as you exhale.

Cat (Fig. 6.21, p. 116)
Do 2–3 times
   Benefits: Improves the flexibility of spine and hands and strengthens the arms and shoulders.
   Precautions: Knee problems or arthritis in the wrists can cause discomfort.
Dog (Fig. 7.5)
Do 2–3 times
   Suggestion: Do this in bare feet—no socks because the feet will slide.

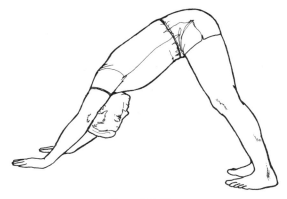

Figure 7.5. Dog.

Benefits: Strengthens arms and shoulders and stretches the legs and back.

Precautions: If you have high blood pressure, do not stay in this pose too long. Do not do if you have glaucoma or retina problems.

Directions

1. Kneeling in the position of the Cat you will then lift the buttocks upward as you inhale.
2. Allow the head to hang down and the back to stretch. Keep the arms straight.
3. Bend the knees slightly to take the stretch off the hamstring muscles at the back of the thigh.
4. Lower yourself down to the kneeling position (Cat).
5. Lift hands off the floor and massage your wrists.

Back Push-up (Fig. 6.20, p. 115)

Benefits: Tones all the muscles from the waist down. Improves flexibility of the shoulders. Helps strengthen the internal muscles (the pubococcygeal) that can help prevent incontinence.

Precautions: Do NOT lift too high if you have neck problems. Instructions are in Chapter 6 (p. 115).

Crocodile Twist (Fig. 6.18, p. 114)

  Benefits: Improves flexibility of the spine, shoulders, hips, waist.

  Precautions: Do not hold your breath during the twisting from side to side.

Pose of Child (Fig. 6.22, p. 117) or **Knees to Chest** (Fig. 6.17, p. 113)

  Benefits: Both gently stretch the back preparing it for the relaxation position which follows.

  Precautions: If you have knee or ankle problems do the Knees to Chest pose.

Relaxation (Fig. 7.6)

5 to 10 min or longer

  Benefits: Stress reduction and release of muscle tension.

  Precautions: You may wish to place a small pillow under your head.

  Hint: If you have a tendency to become cool when you lie down, have a lightweight blanket ready to place over you. This is also a good time to play some "Relaxation," " New Age," or "Classical" music to assist you in your relaxation session.

Directions

1. Begin by sitting on the padded floor or on a mat with the knees bent and feet separated. Remove your glasses.

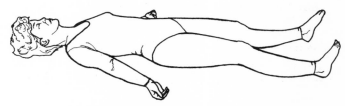

Figure 7.6. Relaxation.

2. Slowly lower the rounded back to the mat, feeling each vertebra touch the floor.

3. If the lower back is comfortable, straighten the legs so that they form the letter "V." You may leave them bent with a pillow under the knees.

4. Place the arms so that the palms are up and about 12 in from the legs.

5. Tuck the shoulders toward the spine, allowing the front of the chest to open more. Keep the shoulders down and away from the ears.

6. Slowly turn the head from side to side to release any tension in the neck. Then bring the head to rest so the nose, center of the mouth, chin, and sternum are in a straight line.

7. The body is now in a position so that no body part has to support another body part, the spine and head are in a straight alignment, and the chest and abdomen are in a position to allow the deep breathing to take place.

8. Please do the following movements to prepare your body to come up from the relaxation session. Keep your eyes closed until after you have done the last step.

    a. Gently stretch the entire body, reaching above your head with your arms and with your thumbs grasping each other.

    b. Turn on to the right side and make a gentle crescent shape with your body as you again stretch, allowing the arms and legs to move behind you so the abdomen can gently stretch.

    c. Flop onto your back like a "rag doll."

    d. Repeat your crescent-shaped stretch on the left side.

    e. Flop again onto your back.

    f. Bend your knees, turn onto your right side, and using your arms slowly push yourself to an upright position.

g. Cross your legs if you are comfortable that way, or leave them straight while you take some deep breaths.

h. Now you will do "palming"—Take your hands and rub your palms together briskly to warm them; then place the palms over your eyes. Open the eyes and look into the darkness of your hands for a few moments, then separate the fingers allowing a little light to enter, and finally take the hands down.

You should now feel very good from your gentle stretching in the Hatha Yoga *asanas*, the breathing, and the relaxation. Some more Hatha Yoga exercises follow—for the eyes.

Eye Exercises

The eyes are moved by muscles, and they too can benefit from exercise. Relaxing exercises of the eyes are included in the practice of yoga, acupuncture, and acupressure. The yoga eye exercises involve movement, while the acupressure approach is through massage. All of these exercises increase the circulation to the eye muscles and can help relieve eyestrain and that tired feeling we sometimes experience.

Instructions for doing some simple eye exercises follow. Seat yourself comfortably and if you wear glasses, remove them. You do not move the head; only the eyes will move. Keep breathing normally and allow the rest of your body to become fully relaxed. These exercises are simple to do and can be done at almost any time or place, except while driving a car. They are especially soothing, however, when you take rest stops during long driving trips. Take just a few moments to do these three brief exercises:

Tracking to the Right and Left

1. Gazing straight in front of you, find a spot to be your center focal point.

2. Slowly and smoothly move the eyes to the right as far as they can go; now move them to the left as far as they can go. Repeat 1 or 2 times.
3. Blink your eyes, then close them to rest.

Tracking up and down
1. Gazing straight in front of you, find a spot to be your center focal point.
2. Slowly and smoothly move the eyes up as far as they will go. (You can probably see the fringe of your hair.) Now slowly and smoothly move them down. (Now you can probably see the side of your nose.) Repeat 1 or 2 times.
3. Blink your eyes, then close them and allow them to rest.

Clock Tracking
1. Gazing straight in front of you, find a spot to be your center focal point; this is where the imaginary hands of the clock are attached.
2. Now, slowly and smoothly move your eyes up to 12 o'clock, then slowly to 1 and 2 o'clock. At 3 o'clock the eyes should be as far to the right as they can go. Then move on to 4 and 5. At 6 o'clock the eyes are looking down. Continue on to 7 and 8. At 9 o'clock the eyes are over to the far left. Move on to 10, 11, and finally 12 o'clock, at which time you are gazing up as far as your eyes can go. Now reverse the movement, moving the eyes to 11, 10, 9, etc.
3. Finish by closing your eyes. Place your palms over them and allow them a few minutes to rest.

As you did these exercises, did you notice a feeling of warmth around the eyes. Did they water? These are common responses because the eyes are probably not used to doing these exercises. Exercising the eyes will not necessarily correct any eye problems, but it is a way of strengthening the muscles and improving circulation. Once you try these exercises you will find they are very refreshing and relaxing.

TAI JI CHUAN

Tai Ji Chuan, or shadow boxing as it has sometimes been called, is also an ancient form of exercise practiced since the 17th century to promote health. In the 1850s, China experienced an interest in this discipline similar to the running boom of the 1960s here in the United States. Today, the form that is most popular, widely taught, and practiced throughout the world is the 24-step simplified Taiji Quan, which was designed by the Chinese government in 1956. It is always done in a peaceful, gentle style. The longer, more complicated forms trace their origins to the martial arts (Wushu).

To learn Tai Ji, it is recommended that you take classes from a trained instructor or practice with a videotape. It is difficult to learn the routine from photos and books, because the essential ingredient, movement from one pose to another, is not present.

The Chinese believe that whoever practices Tai Ji regularly will have the pliability of a child, the vitality of a lumberjack, and the peace of mind of a sage. Research has found that when Tai Ji is performed there is an increase in flexibility. Tai Ji has also been researched as a form of "rhythmic, continuous aerobic activity" and has been designated "moderate" exercise, with the body's consumption of oxygen at 40% to 50% of its maximum. This is a desirable level for the older adult, as has been previously discussed. Another benefit comes from the intense amount of concentration required to do the routine with all the corrections for proper alignment. These slow and gentle movements represent an effort to train the mind as well as the body.

FELDENKRAIS AWARENESS THROUGH MOVEMENT

Moshe Feldenkrais was an innovative man who developed a system of exercises that is easy to learn and is designed to release the habitual movement patterns of the nervous system and help develop improved functioning. The result is better posture, greater ease of movement, increased flexibility, and stress reduction. The technique of body–brain mechanics has been taught throughout the world since Feldenkrais began to develop this system around 1942. As an engineer, both mechanical and electrical, and as a physicist he earned a doctorate in science from the Sorbonne in Paris. In 1947 his first book was published, *Body and Mature Behavior: A Study of Anxiety, Sex, Gravitation and Learning*, which incorporates his academic knowledge and his experiences from yoga, judo, and sports.

Two basic groups of people respond especially well to the work of Feldenkrais: (1) those who have physical problems such as cerebral palsy and multiple sclerosis, pain, or injuries to the neuromuscular system; and (2) those who are involved at a high performance level with their bodies, such as musicians, athletes, dancers, and actors.

The Feldenkrais Technique is most suitable for the older adult as well. The exercises are nonstrenuous and are done as slowly as possible, with no strain or pain. This is because as you become stronger and more flexible, you learn to use your body more effectively. Many of the movements are very small and controlled. Feldenkrais believes that the more completely you make use of your entire muscular system, the more you are aware of the movements and the more the brain is activated. The activated regions then activate adjacent areas, thus increasing the function of the whole brain.

Many of the exercises are done lying down so that the impact of gravity on the body is lessened. An inward sensing of how it feels to do the movement is encouraged. You remain in a state of attention, monitoring your muscular response. You are replacing old movement habits by choice, and assisting the nervous system to develop further. The exercises are done only in a range of movement that is comfortable for each individual.

Although you can work on the exercises at home, it is recommended that you learn with a person who has been trained in the Feldenkrais technique. A list of practitioners can be obtained by writing to the address of the Feldenkrais Guild, listed in the Resource section. Many audiotape lessons are available for at-home practice, with the instructions by Dr. Feldenkrais and also by people he has trained. These range from a single introductory tape costing approximately $15.00 to a series of ten 30-min lessons for $125.00.

The following description will give you an idea of what a Feldenkrais lesson with Jean Houston (protege of Feldenkrais and author) is like. The author, Albert Rosenfeld, shared his experience in an article in the Smithsonian Magazine:

> Vivid use of the imagination is an important part of the Feldenkrais method. I remember doing what seemed at the time a silly exercise. I was sprawled on the ground, face down, with arms and legs spread-eagled. I was told to imagine that I had a continuous groove running all the way from the tip of my left hand, down my arm, then running from my left shoulder diagonally across my back down to my right buttock, then down my right leg to the heel. (Later, the imaginary groove ran from my right hand to my left heel.) Then I was asked to imagine a tiny steel ball that I was to propel along the entire length of the groove through the use of whatever muscles I wished—only I was not to get up or to move my arms from the spread-eagle position. I can tell you that, in concentrating on this activity, I underwent a lot of unfamiliar sensations and exercised a host of tiny muscles I didn't even know I had. And that is part of the Feldenkrais idea.
>
> (Rosenfeld, 1981)

These movement experiences of Feldenkrais can greatly increase your awareness of yourself, your ease of movement, and your self-image. The following is a sample of some of the Feldenkrais movements for you to try: First, sit erect and simply cross your arms in the manner in which you always do. Now glance down and see how your arms and hands are arranged. Next, close your eyes and uncross your arms, then cross them again so they are in the mirror-image arrangement as before. Notice your body's response. Does it feel different to you? You have just done a "habitual movement" the first time and a "nonhabitual movement" the second time. Now we would like for you to try the following two exercises.

Back Lying Arm Movement

1. Starting Position (Fig. 7.7): Lying on your back, make a box with your arms over your chest. Your hands are on opposing elbows. Very slowly do the following:
2. Move the arms from side to side, noticing the reaction as you go to each side. Is there a difference? Do this a number of times (at least 8 to 10). Before you continue, rest your arms for a moment if they are tired.
3. This time move the arms as before but also turn the head so that when the arms go to the right side, the head also turns to the right (Fig. 7.8). Turn back slowly and continue in a smooth movement to the left side. Repeat this a number of times (8 to 10). Notice how the addition of the

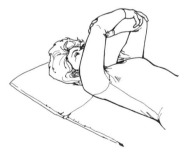

Figure 7.7. Feldenkrais box with arms.

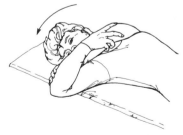

Figure 7.8. Feldenkrais box with arms and head turned to same side.

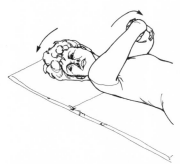

Figure 7.9. Feldenkrais box with arms and head turned to opposite sides.

head movement has changed the body's response. Be aware.

4. This time, as the arms do the same movement, the head turns to the opposite side, so that when the arms are slowly moving over to the right, the head is slowly turning to the left (Fig. 7.9). Try to time the movements to be synchronized so that you reach your maximum range of movement with the arms at the same moment your head has turned as far as it can go comfortably. (Remember, no

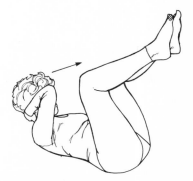

Figure 7.10. Back lying head lift toward knee.

forcing.) Now, notice how the body has reacted to this additional movement.

Back Awareness

1. Starting position: Lie on your back with your arms at your sides, palms down. Notice where your body is contacting the floor and where it is not. Slide a hand under the small of the back to see how high the arch is. It is best to do this on a firm surface without padding; lying on a mattress or bed will not give you the feedback from your body.
2. Gently turn your head from side to side and notice whether there is any tension in either side of your neck.
3. Bend both knees and bring them toward the chest. Place the left hand on the left leg just below the knee. With your right palm lift up your head, and aim your right elbow toward your left knee (Fig. 7.10). Lower your head and then repeat. Now lower your feet to the floor near your buttocks, with your knees remaining bent.
4. On the right side you are only going to think about doing the same routine. So, follow the instructions in Step 3 in your mind only. Do not move the physical body at all. Do this mental practice a second time.
5. Now straighten the legs and notice how the body is in contact with the floor. Try to slide your hand under the small of the back to see if there is a difference.
6. Slowly roll over to your side, coming up on your knees and then stand up. Walk around and notice how you feel.

Feldenkrais believed that we can, with the conscious brain, instruct the body to function at a level much closer to its full potential. He believed that through awareness we can learn to move "with astonishing lightness and freedom," no matter what our age, thus improving the quality of our lives physically, of course, but also intellectually, emotionally, and spiritually (Rosenfeld, 1987).

MASSAGE THERAPY

The beginnings of massage can be traced back to the Greek period when athletes, who were especially favored, were among the first to enjoy the physical and mental benefits of it. The biggest contribution to the field of massage after the Greeks was by the Swedish therapist Per Henrick Ling, who in the early 1900s developed the percussion movements that we now call Swedish massage.

Massage today is not only for the athlete; its benefits can be appreciated and enjoyed by all of us. Trained and certified massage therapists can help restore the function of muscles and joints, improve circulation, aid in the relief of physical fatigue, and assist in stress reduction. They are also trained to use heat, ultrasound, and water therapy to assist in the improvement of joint and muscle function. Some people are at risk of developing blood clots with massage, and it is important to keep this in mind when giving or receiving a massage. Choose a therapist who is a graduate of a recognized, licensed, and approved school of massage. A list of approved schools can be obtained from the National Education Committee of the American Massage Therapy Association. See the Resources section for information on locating a registered, certified massage therapist.

You can massage your own feet, hands, and lower legs, and to some extent even your arms, shoulders, and trunk. Many people find a foot massage to be wonderfully relaxing. Instructions for giving yourself a foot massage follow in the next section.

Basic Foot Massage Instructions

1. Sit and place your foot on your knee, if this position is comfortable, or stand and prop the foot being massaged on the edge of a chair if you have good balance. Better still, put your foot on the lap of a friend.

2. Use a small amount of vegetable oil or lotion, as this allows your hands to glide over the skin with less friction.

3. As you massage, do not pick your hands up repeatedly and then put them back down. When you do this, your body and sensory nerves have to keep making the adjustment. It is best to maintain contact, with at least one hand, with the area being massaged. This is also more soothing.

Massaging the Whole Foot

Gently apply pressure, then squeeze and release, moving your hands all over the foot (Fig. 7.11).

Massaging the Center of Foot

Place your middle finger in the center of the bottom of the foot (near the ball of the foot) and press in, counting to ten and then releasing (Fig. 7.12).

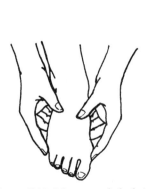

Figure 7.11. Massage whole foot.

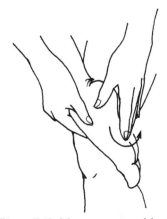

Figure 7.12. Massage center of foot.

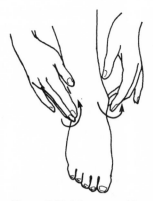

Figure 7.13. Massage ankles.

Massaging the Ankles

Pressing slightly, make small circles above and below and circling the anklebone (Fig. 7.13).

Massaging the Toes

1. Rub each toe for a moment. Then holding the tip of the toe, gently rotate it, and then reverse the direction (Fig. 7.14).
2. Before releasing the toe, pull it to gently stretch it.

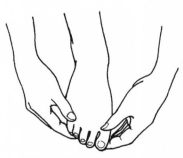

Figure 7.14. Massage toes.

Finish by massaging the whole foot once again and then repeat the massage on the other foot.

RELAXATION AND STRESS REDUCTION TECHNIQUES

Hatha Yoga, Tai Ji Chuan, and Feldenkrais awareness through movement techniques, which have previously been discussed, are all holistic approaches to bodywork that involve controlled breathing and stress reduction along with the exercising. This section will now expand and discuss other stress-reduction techniques.

Progressive Relaxation (Jacobson Relaxation Technique)

Over thirty years ago Dr. Edmond Jacobson was one of the first Americans to study the relationship between muscle contraction, relaxation, and the response of the nerves. The first step in progressive relaxation involves learning to recognize that muscle tension is present by consciously and deliberately contracting the muscles and noticing the exertion and the discomfort present, followed by their absence when the muscles are allowed to go limp and to totally relax. The second step is learning to relax completely: first, the body's large muscles (legs, arms, trunk, and neck), followed by the smaller muscles of the face, eyes, and throat. Dr. Jacobson's book, *You Must Relax,* was first published in 1957, and has served as the basis for the Western world's approach to and acceptance of relaxation training.

Breathing Exercises

Deep breathing exercises can also calm the body. One of the reasons is that with the mind concentrating on the breath moving in and out, it cannot be thinking of other things that may be stressful. Some recommend that you sit or lie down, with eyes closed, and inhale slowly through the nose and exhale slowly through the mouth. Repeat this 8–10 times; then breathe normally and stay in your relaxed state for awhile.

In yoga, the alternate-nostril breath, one of the pranayama (breathing) techniques, is also taught to calm the body. This technique involves inhaling through one nostril, then exhaling through the other side; then inhaling on that side and exhaling through the nostril where you began (Fig. 7.15). To begin, you should sit with eyes closed, spine erect, and head centered and level. Place your index finger on the bridge of your nose, with the thumb controlling the opening and closing of one nostril and the middle and ring finger controlling the other nostril. Check the flow of air in each nostril first, and begin the inhalation on the side that is most open. Inhale to a count of 4, 6, or 8 (whichever is most comfortable for your lung capacity), and exhale on the same count but through the other nostril. Then complete the round by inhaling on that side and exhaling on the side where you began. Repeat this cycle for a total of 5 or 6 times. Then take a normal deep breath and lie back or sit quietly to enjoy the calm feeling you have created for yourself.

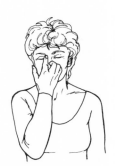

Figure 7.15. Alternate nostril breath.

Herbert Benson, a Harvard Medical School cardiologist wrote a book, *The Relaxation Response*, which was a best-seller in 1975. The technique he presents combines deep breathing with relaxation. He recommends doing the breathing for 20–30 min twice a day.

Meditation

This is not as mysterious or difficult to do as some people think. It simply involves sitting quietly, breathing deeply, and concentrating on a single word or image for 15–20 min. The secret is concentration. If your mind wanders or begins thinking, just bring it back directly to the word or image or to the breathing. Buddhists practice this type of meditation, as do the followers of the Maharishi Mahesh Yogi, who popularized the Transcendental Meditation system from Yoga. It has been reported in more than 700 studies that "TM" can reduce tension, blood pressure, and levels of certain hormones.

Visualization, Music, and Imagery

The connection between the brain and body is becoming more widely recognized. It is being discussed in popular magazines and also researched in respected centers of learning such as Harvard, Yale, and Duke Universities. The applications of this emerging field of study range from simply practicing positive thinking to the intense mental practice used by Olympic athletes of all ages and countries to perfect their skills. There are many ways that the "interconnectedness theory" can enhance the lives of anyone—older adults included.

Anyone can benefit from mental practice if, in their daily lives, they allow some time to develop this technique. Perhaps, it may involve learning a new skill such as typing or the use of computers, practicing "walking in your mind" following reconstructive hip surgery, or perfecting a tennis or golf swing. This technique is also part of the approach taken in the many self-healing programs and books that have appeared in recent years. The Simontons, Bernard Siegal, and Norman Cousins have all made use of this approach, and similar ones, to help people in situations of chronic pain and terminal illness.

Using the imagination, with soft, gentle music (see the Resources section) playing in the background can help some people to relax. Creating in your mind's eye a place where you have felt peaceful (for example, walking on a beach with the sounds of ocean waves and seagulls chirping, the warm sun, a gentle wind) can be very effective in bringing about a relaxed feeling.

Flotation Tanks

Although not for everybody, these vinyl or fiberglass tanks, which are totally enclosed and filled with a solution of water and epsom salts, are gaining in popularity. In one of these tanks you are in a state of sensory deprivation; alone, in a totally dark environment, with only the sound of your own breathing. The length of stay in a tank is usually 1 hr. With the high salt concentration making you buoyant, you learn to relax and let the water support you. Many people find it an interesting and refreshing experience. (It is also possible to leave the door open, for those who are uncomfortable with it closed.)

Additional Suggestions for Mastering Stress

Daily living can be stressful for all of us, no matter what our age. Try incorporating the following eleven steps into your life to bring about a calmer response to the large and small stressors we all encounter from time to time.

1. Do something that you love to do each day.
2. Say no when you really don't want to do something.
3. Exercise every day.
4. Take many deep, slow breaths during the day.
5. Smile often, and others will smile back.
6. Let your forehead and eyes be relaxed and soft, no frowning.
7. Monitor your intake of caffeine, sugar, salt, and alcohol.
8. Don't be too demanding of yourself.
9. Associate with people you trust and feel at ease with; those who bolster you up rather than drag you down.
10. Love yourself.
11. Laugh!

BIBLIOGRAPHY

References

Bell, L., and Seyfer, E., 1982, *Gentle Yoga*, Cedar Rapids, Iowa, Ingram Press.

Benson, H., and Klipper, M. Z., 1979, *The Relaxation Response*, New York, Avon Books.

Birkel, D. A., 1991, *Hatha Yoga: Developing Body, Mind and Inner Self*, Dubuque, Iowa, Eddie Bowers Publishing, Inc.

Cousins, N., 1983, *The Healing Heart: Antidotes to Panic and Helplessness*, New York, W. W. Norton Publishers.

Cousins, N., 1989, *Head First: The Biology of Hope*, New York, E. P. Dutton.

Dunn, T., 1987, The practice and spirit of T'ai Chi Ch'uan, *Yoga Journal* 77:62–65, 90–91, 94.

Houston, J., 1982, *The Possible Human: A Course in Extending Your Physical, Mental, and Creative Abilities*, Los Angeles, J. P. Tarcher.

Jacobson, E., 1976, *You Must Relax*, 5th ed., New York, McGraw-Hill.

Rosenfeld, A., 1981, Teaching the body how to program the brain is Moshe's miracle, *Smithsonian* **11**(10):52–56, 58–59.

Siegal, B., 1986, *Love, Medicine and Miracles*, New York, Harper & Row.

Suggested Reading

Ardell, D., 1979, *High Level Wellness*, New York, Bantam Books.

Benson, H., 1987, Beyond relaxation—The renewable mind, *American Health— Fitness of Body and Mind* **6**(7):76–83.

Benson, H., and Proctor, W., 1987, *Your Maximum Mind*, New York, N.Y. Times Books.

Borysenko, J., 1987, Visions to boost immunity, *American Health—Fitness of Body and Mind* **6**(6):56–61

Brosnan, B., and Brosnan, C. B., 1982, *Yoga for Handicapped People*, London, Souvenir Press (E & A) Ltd.

Christensen, A., and Rankin, D., 1975, *Easy Does It Yoga for Older People*, New York, Harper and Row.

Chuungliang, A. C., 1987, *Embrace Tiger, Return to Mountain*, Berkeley, Calif., Celestial Arts.

Crooks, C., 1985, Can a Mineral Mitigate Stress? *American Health—Fitness of Body and Mind* **4**(5):112.

Ewehock, G., and Sieapany, C., *Ten Minutes to Health*, P.O. Box 20850, Reno, Nev. 84515, CRCS Publications.

Feldenkrais, M., 1977, *Awareness through Movement*, New York, Harper & Row.

Feldenkrais, M., 1981, *The Elusive Obvious*, Cupertino, Calif., Meta Publications.

Feldenkrais, M., 1986, *The Master Moves*, Cupertino, Calif., Meta Publications.

Folan, L., 1981, *Yoga and Your Life*, New York, Macmillan Publishing Co., Inc.

Friedman, M., and Rosenman, R. H., 1974, *Type A Behavior and Your Heart*, New York, Knopf Publishing Co.

Freidman, M., and Chungliang, A. H., 1989, A master of moving meditation, *New Realities* **9**(3):10–20.

Holmes, B., 1984, Moving well with Feldenkrais, *Yoga Journal* **54**:30–32.

Iyengar, B. K. S., 1985, *The Concise Light on Yoga*, New York, Schockon Books.

Larronde, S., 1982, Lessons in living, *Modern Maturity* **33**(3):61–62.

Levey, J., 1987, *The Fine Arts of Relaxation, Concentration, and Meditation: Ancient Skills for Modern Minds*, London, Wisdom Publications.

Maxwell-Hudson, C., 1987, *The Complete Book of Massage*, New York, Random House.

Ornish, D., Dr. Dean Ornish's guide to a healthy heart, *Yoga Journal* **97**:50–53, 106–107.

Pelletier, K.R., 1977, *Mind as Healer, Mind as Slayer: A Holistic Approach to Preventing Stress Disorders*, New York, Dell Books.

Perry, P., 1986, Grasp the bird's tail, *American Health—Fitness of Body and Mind* **5**(1):58–63.

Selye, H., 1974, *Stress Without Distress*, Philadelphia, Lippincott.

Simonton, C. J., and Simonton, S., 1978, *Getting Well Again: A Step-by-Step Guide to Overcoming Cancer for Patients and Their Families*, Los Angeles, J. P. Tarcher.

Wei, L., Reid, L. M., Taijiquan: an adaptable Chinese exercise program, *Journal of Physical Education Recreation and Dance* **60**(3):77–79.

Resources

Magazines

American Health—Fitness of Body and Mind, American Health Partners, 80 Fifth Ave., New York, NY 10011.

Nutrition Action Newsletter, Center for Science in the Public Interest, 1501 16th St., N.W., Washington, D.C. 20036.

Yoga Journal, 2054 University Ave., Berkeley, CA 94704-9975.

Audiotapes

Moshe Feldenkrais for the Older Citizen. Series of ten 30-minute lessons to be done sitting in a chair or lying down. Includes tapes, instructions in vinyl binder, and *Learn To Learn* booklet. Order from: ATM Recordings, 1429 Montague Street, N.W., Washington, D.C. 20011. (Also suitable for anyone whose movements are impaired because of accident, disease, or disuse.)

Della Grotte, J., P.O. Box 612, Westminster, MA 01473. Write for information on current Feldenkrais tapes and prices.

Holmes, B.T., *The Feldenkrais Lessons: Awareness Through Movement*. Twelve 90-min tapes. Order from: Haven Corporation, 802 Madison Ave., Dept J8, Evanston, IL 60202.

Videos

Massage Videos

Massage Your Mate, Ozman, Inc., 596-A Hudson St., #K-17, New York, NY 10004,
    Telephone: (212)620-3832.
Massage for Health, Healing Arts Home Video, P.O. Box 708, Northbrook, IL 60065.

Tai Ji Videotapes

Wayfarer Publications, Dept. YG, P.O. Box 26156, Los Angeles, CA 90026.
Interarts, Dept. H., 1283 S. LaBrea Ave., Suite 162, Los Angeles, CA 90019.

Organizations

American Massage and Therapy Association, James Bowling, Executive Secretary/
    Treasurer, P.O. Box 1270, 310 Cherokee Street, Kingsport, TN, Telephone: (615)
    245-8071.
Feldenkrais Guild, P.O. Box 111145, San Francisco, CA 94101. Write for information
    on current tapes and prices.
Tai Ji Association, P.O. Box 56113, Atlanta, GA 30343. Write for a directory of
    teachers.

Music

Catalogs

Halpern Sounds, Suite 9, 1775 Old County Road, Belmont, CA 94002.
Windham Hill Productions, Inc., P.O. Box 9388, Stanford, CA 94305, Telephone:
    (415) 329-0647.
Institute for Music, Health and Education, Director, Don G. Campbell, P.O Box
    1244, Boulder, CO 80306.
Heartbeats, from Backroads Distributors, 417 Tamal Plaza, Corte Madera, CA
    94925, Telephone: (800) 825-4848. They offer the Public Radio broadcasts of
    programs from "Hearts in Space."
Heartsong Review, P.O. Box 1084, Cottage Grove, OR 97424. This is published twice a
    year as a resource guide for new-age music as well as a catalog. Two-year
    subscription: $10.00; one-year: $6.00.

Audiotapes

Campbell, D., "Angels," "Crystal Rainbows," "Crystal Meditations," "Cosmic Classics," and "Symphony for the Inner Self."

Enya, "Watermark" and "Enya."

Halpern, S., "Dawn," "Spectrum Suite," "Crystal Suite," and "Gaia's Groove."

Halpern, S., and Kelly, G., "Ancient Echos."

Rowland, M., "The Fairy Ring," "Solace," "Titania," and "Silver Wings."

Solitude Series, Nature Soundtracks: swamps, lakes, oceans.

Environments Series: oceans, meadows, forests, thunderstorm, sailboat, and ocean.

Horn, P., "Inside the Pyramids," "Inside the Taj Mahal," "Peace Album."

Vollenweider, A., "Caverna Magica," "Behind the Garden . . .," "Dancing With the Lion," and "Down to the Moon."

CHAPTER 8

Resistance Training

But to act, that each tomorrow brings us
farther than today.

Longfellow

To see ourselves growing stronger each day is a rewarding and satisfying experience—not only for the highly motivated and fit, but for the frail elderly as well. Resistance training is one way that has been found to bring about a steady increase in strength. Although decrease in muscular strength is known to be part of the normal aging process, research in weight-resistance programs for older adults has shown that muscular strength and muscle mass can be restored to a certain degree.

In a study at the Boston Hebrew Rehabilitation Center for the Aged, ten residents aged 86–96 years did weight lifting on a standard weight-and-pulley system for three days a week for eight weeks, gradually increasing the weight lifted from 15 to

43 lb. At the end of the study the group showed an average strength gain of 174% (Evans *et al.*, 1990). Likewise, a study of 13 men, aged 60–69 years, done at Ball State University, showed that there was a significant increase in lean body weight, meaning that the participants increased their lean muscle. Even though it was previously thought that when muscle strength and muscle mass had been lost there was no way to reverse the process, it is now believed by many that such a reversal is possible with carefully monitored weight-resistance training.

Nevertheless, of all the approaches to exercise for the older adult, resistance training is probably considered by many exercise specialists to be the most controversial. The reason is that the strain of pushing or pulling against the resistance of a weight or a rubberband can cause the blood pressure to rise. This is a potential hazard, then, for those with high blood pressure or cardiovascular disease. Some exercise specialists believe that this pressure in the cardiovascular system can be lessened by correct breathing techniques and we will carefully examine this later in this chapter.

Gains in strength in the frail elderly as well as in those more active can contribute to more independence in living. The use of weight-resistance equipment should be supervised and the response of older persons monitored by those trained in working in exercise with older adults.

It is important to understand the muscle activity during resistance exercises. Remember, *isotonic* exercise is when the muscles are changing length and are moving; this is considered a dynamic activity. *Isometric* exercise is when the muscles are contracted without changing length: this is a static activity. *Isokinetic* exercise is when the muscles are contracting at a constant speed during the full range of movement, and the resistance against the muscle is always present, but varies. The harder you pull or push, the harder the machine resists you. The Nautilus weight machines are of this type, as are the Hydra-Fitness machines, which have a hydraulic cylinder that automatically adjusts to the strength and speed of the individual.

It is also necessary to review the *overload principle* of exercise, which is a basic concept in weight-resistance exercise programs. To increase in strength, the muscle needs to be challenged by being forced to contract at its near-maximum tension level. The amount of weight or resistance is continually and gradually increased in order for the exerciser to gain in strength. Thus, the muscle group is worked a little harder each time. When it can do the work of lifting 8–10 repetitions for two times then more weight is added. This is known as "progressive resistance." Before we go on, two terms commonly used in weight training, "reps" and "sets," need explaining. Reps refers to repetitions. It is recommended that you lift the weight for an exercise, or at each station, 8–10 repetitions. Sets refers to the number of times you complete 8–10 reps or go around to each station. One set is doing each exercise or weight station 8–10 reps one time; two sets means doing each station or exercise a second time. It is possible and safe to do three sets.

BENEFITS OF RESISTANCE TRAINING

1. Muscle strength has been found to decrease as part of the normal aging process. With resistance training on weights, as research has proven, this can be reversed.
2. Improvements in posture often take place because the strengthened muscles can hold the skeletal system in better alignment.
3. For women, working with weights may help prevent osteoporosis, since research has shown that the movement of

muscles and tendons stimulates the bone to become stronger and more dense.

4. It is now known that resistance exercise can increase the lean body tissue: muscles.

PRECAUTIONS

1. Do not hold your breath while exercising. If you keep the windpipe (glottis) open by counting out loud, you prevent the intrathoracic pressure from rising, thus removing a threat to the cardiovascular system.

2. If you do have coronary or artery disease, you should not do isometric or resistive-type exercises alone—only do them with competent supervision.

3. If you miss some days of doing your weight resistance workout, you must either: (1) do fewer repetitions at the weight or exercise you had done the last time; or (2) go back to the next lower weight and do your 8–10 repetitions.

GENERAL GUIDELINES

1. Always do the warm-up and cool-down stretches for all of the muscle groups you are using. See Table 8.1 for a suggested warm-up routine and Table 8.2 for a cool-down routine. Refer to the Basic 40 numbered exercises described in Chapter 6.

Table 8.1
Warm-up Stretches for Resistance Training

#1. Head Turns (p. 100)	#13. Chest Stretch in Doorway (p. 109)
#2. Head Tilts (p. 101)	#30. Lower Leg Stretch at Wall
#5. Single Arms Swings (p. 103)	(p. 123)
#6. Arm Circles (p. 104)	#31. Standing Leg Swings and Circles
#7. Wall Walk and Slide (p. 104)	(p. 124)
#10. Behind the Back Tie Stretch	#32. Tree Balance (p. 125)
(p. 107)	

2. Maintain proper body alignment at all times. Follow the directions to prevent injury.
3. Follow these breathing suggestions: (1) Keep your breath flowing; do not hold it; (2) Inhale; (3) Slowly count out loud to six as you are exerting force against the resistance, you are exhaling as you do this; (4) Release your force against the resistance slowly as you count to six mentally. Inhale back to starting position; (5)Pause and relax, breathing normally (for about six counts); (6) Repeat. Inhale first and then exhale as you move against the resistance following the procedure explained above.

Table 8.2
Cool-down Stretches for Resistance Training

#5. Single Arm Swings (p. 103)	#13. Chest Stretch in Doorway (p. 109)
#6. Arm Circles (p. 104)	#17. Knees to Chest (p. 112)
#7. Wall Walk and Slide (p. 104)	#18. Crocodile Twist (p. 114)
#10. Behind the Back Tie Stretch	#19. Knee overs (p. 114)
(p. 107)	#20. Back Pushup (p. 115)

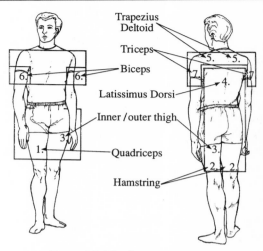

Figure 8.1. Muscle group sequence.

4. Ease off if you are having any pain. If pain persists, stop exercising. You may want to check with your physician.
5. Always do the movements through a complete range of motion without locking the elbows and knees.
6. Do not work the same muscle group two stations in a row. See Fig. 8.1 for the recommended sequence for working the muscle groups.
7. Allow 48 hr between your strength training sessions for the muscles to recover.
8. Don't hesitate to ask questions of those who have experience, especially those of your age.

RESISTANCE TRAINING WITH INNER TUBES AND RUBBER BANDS

An inexpensive way to do resistance-type exercises at home is to use bicycle inner tubes or the new shorter rubber bands that come in different thicknesses and sizes to vary the resistance of the exercise. Inner tubes, being longer, are suitable for doing exercises in a chair or placing under your foot when standing or lying down. They may also be attached to a handle such as a garage door. These inner tubes can usually be obtained at no charge from your local bicycle shop. Wash them and cut in half near the stem (removing the stem since it could scratch you). The other stretch bands can be bought in sporting-goods stores or ordered by mail. See the Resources section at the end of the chapter for addresses.

The guidelines and precautions already mentioned also apply for exercising with inner tubes and bands as well. In addition, read the guidelines that pertain to tubes and bands specifically.

Guidelines for Bands and Tubes

1. The larger the circumference of the tube or band the less the resistance. The bicycle inner tubes can be made smaller by retying the ends to make a smaller circle. Exercise with the amount of resistance that you are comfortable with.
2. Check the bands for tears and holes each time before using them. If a band breaks during exercising you could be injured.
3. Keep the band or inner tube away from your face and do not direct it toward another person.

4. Cover your bare skin where the band is in contact; wear gloves and sweat pants or leg warmers. This will prevent any irritation to the skin and prevent the band/tube from slipping.
5. Do the warm-up (Table 8.1) and cool-down (Table 8.2) routines.

Inner Tube or Rubber Band Workout

Quadriceps (Fig. 8.2)
Directions
1. Sit down. Bending knees, place the shortened tube or band around the left ankle.
2. Anchor the band or tube by stepping on it with the right foot.
3. Lie back and straighten the left leg and inhale as you raise it as high as you can comfortably, and exhale as you lower. Repeat with right leg.
4. Level
    Beginner: Repeat for a total of 8.
    Challenge: Repeat for a total of 12.

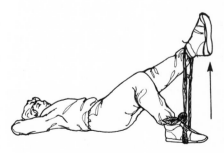

Figure 8.2. Quadriceps.

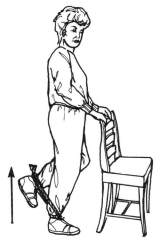

Figure 8.3. Hamstrings.

Hamstrings (Fig. 8.3)

Directions

1. Stand facing the back of a chair and hold on for balance.
2. A shortened tube or a band is around both ankles. Keep knees together and do not let the back arch. Inhale.
3. Bend the left knee and, keeping the foot flexed, exhale as you curl the lower leg toward the buttocks drawing the heel closer to the body. Inhale as you lower to starting.
4. Do your repetitions and then repeat with the right leg.
5. Level

   Beginner: Repeat for a total of 8.

   Challenge: Repeat for a total of 12.

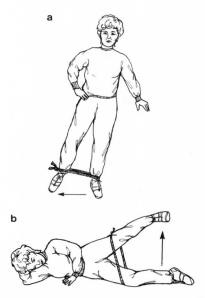

Figure 8.4. (a) Outer thigh, standing and (b) outer thigh, lying.

Outer Thigh, Standing and Lying (Fig. 8.4)

A. Standing (Fig. 8.4a)

   Directions

   1. Stand with your left side to a chair and hold on to the back for balance.

   2. The shortened tube or a band is around both ankles. Inhale.

   3. Exhale as you lift the right leg (outside leg) as far as possible to the side and inhale as you return to the starting position.

   4. Do your repetitions, turn around and repeat with the left leg.

B. Lying (Fig. 8.4b)

   Directions

   1. Lie on your right side and let your arms support you.

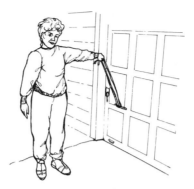

Figure 8.5. Deltoids.

2. The shortened tube or a band is around both legs just above your knees. Inhale.
3. Exhale as you lift your straight left leg up. Keep your pelvis facing forward. Inhale as you lower to starting position.
4. Do your repetitions, turn to the left side and repeat with the right leg lifting.
5. Level
   Beginner: Repeat for a total of 8.
   Challenge: Repeat for a total of 12.

Deltoids (Fig. 8.5)
Directions
1. Stand and anchor the long tube, or two bands joined, under the right foot or attach to an immovable object such as a garage door. Inhale.
2. Holding the other end of the tube, exhale and lift the straight right arm out to the side as high as you can. Inhale as you lower to starting position.
3. Maintain an erect posture and do not sway.
4. Do your repetitions and then repeat with the left arm.
5. Level
   Beginner: Repeat for a total of 8.
   Challenge: Repeat for a total of 12.

Lower Legs, Flex and Point (Fig. 8.6)

Directions

1. Sit on the floor leaning back on hands and arms. Right leg is straight and left leg is bent with the heel by the right knee.
2. The shortened tube or band is anchored at the ball of the right foot. The band is around the top of the left foot. Inhale.
3. Exhale as you flex (pull the toes of the left foot) toward the body and release and inhale.
4. Do your repetitions, and then repeat with the right foot.
5. Level

    Beginner: Repeat for a total of 8.

    Challenge: Repeat for a total of 12.

Shoulder Raises (Fig. 8.7)

Directions

1. Stand with the inner tube or two bands joined together and anchored under your right foot.

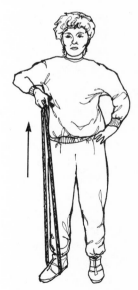

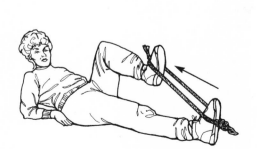

Figure 8.6. Lower leg, flex and point.   Figure 8.7. Shoulder raises.

2. Hold the other end in the right hand with the arm extended down by your thigh. Inhale.
3. Exhale as you bend your elbow, bringing your arm up to the level of your shoulder. Inhale as you lower arm slowly to side.
4. Do your repetitions, and then repeat with the left arm.
5. Level
   Beginner: Repeat for a total of 8.
   Challenge: Repeat for a total of 12.

Biceps Curl (Fig. 8.8)
Directions
1. Stand with the shortened tube or a band held in both hands.
2. Bend right arm and anchor at waist level with fist up.
3. Left hand is fist down with the arm extended downward and the elbow relaxed. Inhale.
4. Exhale as you curl the right arm toward the chest and do not allow the left arm to move. Inhale as you return to starting position.
5. Do your repetitions, and then repeat with the left arm.
6. Level
   Beginner: Repeat for a total of 8.
   Challenge: Repeat for a total of 12.

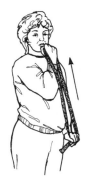

Figure 8.8. Biceps curl.

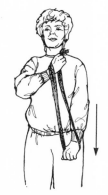

Figure 8.9. Triceps press.

Triceps Press (Fig. 8.9)

Directions

1. Stand with the shortened tube or a band held in both hands.
2. Right hand is placed palm toward chest near clavicle.
3. Left hand is bent at waist level holding band with palm down. Inhale.
4. Exhale as you press the left hand down toward floor. Do not lock elbow. Return to starting position.
5. Do your repetitions and then repeat with the right arm.
6. Level
   Beginner: Repeat for a total of 8.
   Challenge: Repeat for a total of 12.

Now remember to do your cool-down stretches.

MACHINE RESISTANCE TRAINING

If you have access to a gym or a weight room and would enjoy a challenge of working with machines please read further. Keeping in mind the precautions and general guidelines discussed, refer now to the following guidelines specific for working on machines.

Guidelines for Machines

1. It is best to begin a weight-resistance program on machines under the supervision of a knowledgeable instructor who has had experience helping others of your age.
2. When you are working with the weight machines always do your workout in the presence of others. If at home invite a friend over to participate with you.
3. To find your starting weight for each station at the machine, estimate the heaviest amount you think you can lift one time and try it. If that is your "maximum" weight, you can then take 60% to 70% of that weight. For instance, if you can lift 40 lb on the bench press one time, then take 60% to 70% of 40 lb, which is 24–28 lbs, and that is your starting weight. Weight machines are usually in increments of 5–10 lb so you would start at 25 or 30 in this example.
4. It is important to record the weight lifted, the number of repetitions at each station, and how many sets you did. Also record how you felt (tired or strong), and check off that you did your warm-up and cool-down stretches. See Appendix K for a form to use in recording your data.

You are now ready to begin your program on the machines. Refer again to Fig. 8.1 to follow the sequence of working the larger muscle groups first and ending with the smaller muscle groups. The following workout has the stations and exercises in sequence to correspond with the muscle groups in Fig. 8.1.

General Conditioning Resistance Training Program

Now you are ready to begin your exercise session on the machines. This suggested work-out is designed for the Universal machines. Do one or two sets of 5–10 repetitions each.

Quadriceps (Fig. 8.10)
Directions
1. Sit on the bench with both feet under the rollers. Do not lie back. Inhale.
2. Exhale as you extend your legs, but do not lock the knees.

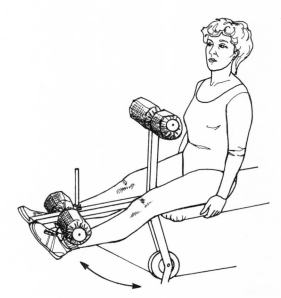

Figure 8.10. Quadriceps.

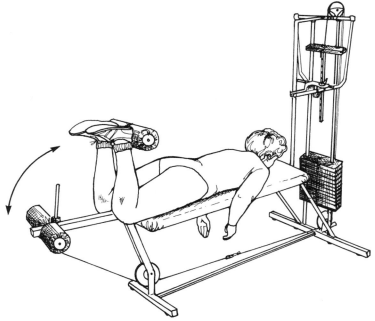

Figure 8.11. Hamstrings.

3. Hold for 1 sec and inhale as you return to the starting position.

Hamstrings (Fig. 8.11)

Directions

1. Lie face down on the bench and hook both heels under the rollers. Inhale.
2. Exhale as you pull rollers up to 90° (or near) and hold for 6 sec and inhale as you return to starting position.

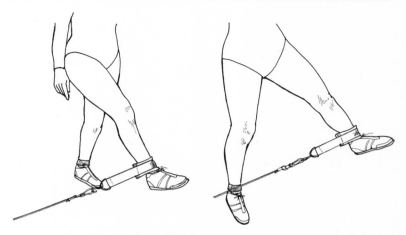

Figure 8.12. Leg crossovers.

Leg Crossovers (Fig. 8.12)
Directions
1. Attach strap to biceps station.
2. Stand with your side to the weights and put one foot through the strap. Inhale.
3. Exhale as you pull the leg across body (Fig. 8.12a).
4. Turn other side to weights. Inhale and exhale as you push the leg away from body (Fig. 8.12b).
5. Keep the leg straight.
6. Now repeat with the other leg.

Lat Bar (Fig. 8.13)
Directions
1. Grip bar on handles and pull down until you are kneeling. You can also do this sitting in a chair or on a bench. Inhale.
2. From the position you have chosen, exhale as you pull the bar down in front until you reach shoulder level.
3. Inhale as you extend the arms and exhale as you pull the bar down in back of your head to shoulder level.

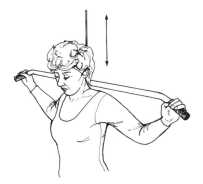

Figure 8.13. Lat bar.

Bench Press (Fig. 8.14)

Directions

1. Lie on bench, head next to the machine.
2. The handles should be lined up approximately with the shoulders.
3. Place your feet flat on the bench, with knees bent. Inhale.
4. Exhale as you lift to extension, but don't lock elbows. Inhale and lower.

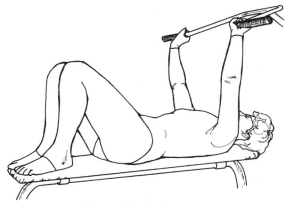

Figure 8.14. Bench press.

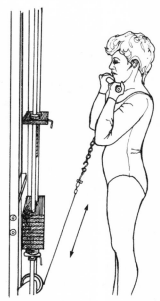

Figure 8.15. Biceps curl.

Biceps Curl (Fig. 8.15)

Directions

1. Stand facing the weights.
2. Hold the bar with both hands, palms up. Inhale.
3. Exhale as you flex your arms until the bar meets your shoulders.
4. Inhale as you return to starting position.
5. Make sure you keep your back straight.

Triceps Press (Fig. 8.16)

Directions

1. Stand facing the lat bar, with palms facing down.
2. Grasp the bar so that your hands are shoulder-width apart. Inhale.
3. Exhale as you pull down to extension and return.

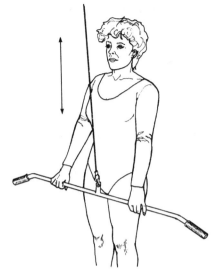

Figure 8.16. Triceps press.

Remember to follow this workout with the cool-down stretches recommended in Table 8.2.

SUMMARY

It is very important in weight-resistance exercises to record your weight lifted, the repetitions, and the number of sets. It is also very important to increase gradually using the "Overload Principle." Now that you have become familiar with one of the more strenuous forms of exercise, you may want to look in the next chapter for information on planning a walking program.

BIBLIOGRAPHY

References

Fiatarone, M., Marks, E. C., Ryan, N. D., Meredith, C. N., Lipsitz, L. A., and Evans, E. W. J., 1990, High-intensity strength training in nonagenarians: Effects on skeletal muscle, *Journal of American Medical Association* **263**: 3029–3034.

Rikkers, R., 1986, *Seniors on the Move*, Champaign, Illinois, Human Kinetics Publishers, Inc.

Spackman, R. R., 1981, *Conditioning for Senior Citizens*, Carbondale, Illinois, Hillcrest House, pp. 12–14.

Sullivan, M., 1987, Atrophy and exercise, *Journal of Gerontological Nursing* **13**(7): 26–31.

Equipment

Dyna-Bands, Future Dynamics, Inc., 3064 West Degerton, Silver Lake, OH 49224, Telephone: 1 (800) 537-5512.

Pumping Rubber, SPRI Products, Inc., 507 North Wolf Road, Wheeling, IL 60090, Telephone: 1 (800) 222-7774

Suggested Readings

Becque, M. D., 1989, *Effects of 12 weeks of Hydraulic Resistance Training on Body Composition, Strength, and Walking Performance of Older Males*, Microform Publications, College of Human Development and Perfomance, University of Oregon, Eugene, Ore.

Fiatarone, M., 1990, Pumping iron helps granny too, *Science News* **137**:398.

Work, J. A., 1989, Strength training: A bridge to independence for the elderly, *The Physician and Sports Medicine* **17**(1):134–136, 138, 140.

CHAPTER 9
Walking

Walking is man's best medicine.
Hippocrates

More and more people are finding walking to be a pleasant, inexpensive, and sociable way to enjoy the benefits of regular exercise. It can be done almost anywhere, indoors or out, with little cost for equipment and virtually no risk to health. Just remember to follow the basic exercise guidelines regarding warm-up and cool-down routines found in Chapter 6 and those related to weather in Chapter 4. If you decide to walk you will have lots of company. There are now about 54 million exercise walkers in this country and the number of new walkers is increasing every month.

It does not take a great deal of strength or stamina to begin a walking program. Even if you have been ill or totally sedentary, you can begin by walking for 1–2 min, resting a minute, and repeating this until you begin to feel tired. Gradually you will see your strength and stamina increase. If you are beginning your

Table 9.1
Modified Walking Program for Senior Adults

Exercise period	Miles	Level I (pace: ¼ mile in 5 min, or 1 mile in 20 min.)	Level II (pace: ¼ mile in 4 min, or 1 mile in 16 min.)	Level III (pace: ¼ mile in 3½ min, or 1 mile in 14 min.)
1 and 2	1	20	16	14
3 and 4	1¼	25	20	17½
5 and 6	1½	30	24	21
7 and 8	1¾	35	28	24½
9 and 10	2	40	32	28
11 and 12	2¼	45	36	31½
13 and 14	2½	50	40	35
15 and 16	2¾	55	44	38½
17 and 18	3	60	48	42

walking program in a healthier state, try walking for 20 min four or five times a week. Then, you can begin to follow the walking program outlined in Table 9.1, moving from one level to another as your strength and speed increase and when you experience no discomfort after two consecutive days at a given level. Begin the program by measuring a one-mile route in your neighborhood, over safe and pleasant terrain. Walk this route regularly, then increase the distance when you feel you are ready. If you prefer to walk indoors, many shopping malls are now opening their doors early to accomodate the new group of exercisers known as "mall walkers." This is a pleasant way to exercise in safety and regardless of extremes in weather, either alone or with friends.

WALKING TECHNIQUES

Although walking may seem like the most natural thing in the world, there are some techniques to help you walk more efficiently

(Fig. 9.1). The following suggestions will also help you break any bad walking habits you may have developed.

1. Remember to maintain an erect posture with your head and chest up and your abdominal muscles contracted slightly (that means the muscles are tightened and pulled in, but not uncomfortably so). Walking with a bean bag on your head or with a dowel stick held behind your head and resting lightly on your shoulders (Fig. 9.2) will help you develop this good posture.

2. Allow the arms to swing naturally, with the opposite arm and leg moving forward simultaneously.

3. Inhale and exhale deeply and rhythmically.

4. Set a pace fast enough to be comfortable but not so fast as to leave you breathless. You should be able to carry on a conversation with a companion. If you find you are breathing too fast or too hard, slow the pace down a bit.

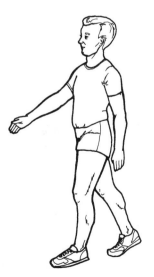

Figure 9.1. Walking technique.

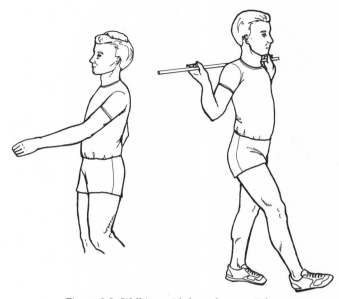

Figure 9.2. Walking with bean bag or stick.

5. Begin the movement of the stride at the hip.
6. Keep your feet 2–4 in apart with both pointing forward, not turned in or out.
7. Place the heel first, and then roll forward to push off the ball of the foot and big toe. Do not walk only on the ball of the foot or "flat-footed," because this can cause an injury or muscle soreness.
8. When walking rapidly either up or down an incline, lean forward slightly.

Many cities and towns, even small ones, have set up walking programs in which you follow an already-delineated walking course. In addition, the Rockport walking test, described in Chapter 2, and the program developed by the Rockport Shoe Company (see Resources for address) are gaining in popularity and are being used widely throughout the country.

EQUIPMENT

The equipment needed for walking (clothing and shoes) is minimal and has already been discussed in Chapter 4. Shoes are the major consideration and virtually the only expense in a walking program, so try to get the best shoe you can, even if it seems expensive initially. A good walking shoe will last for years and will save much wear and tear on your feet. If you have joint problems at the knees, hips, or ankles, or if you have a tendency to develop shinsplints (painful strain of the muscles at the front of the lower leg), you may want to try using an insert to absorb some of the force generated as your foot strikes the ground when you run or walk. If you think these might help, try on the walking shoes with the inserts in place to assure a proper fit and to make sure that there is ample room in the toe box.

You may enjoy using a pedometer to convert the number of your steps into miles, and a walking stick or staff can provide a wonderful physical and psychological support. Always carry identification as well as the name of a friend or family member who may be called in an emergency. Carry some change in case you need to make a phone call yourself. These precautions are important not only for older adults but for all exercisers.

Some walkers enjoy walking to music using a small portable radio or tape player with headphones. This helps you keep time with the music and walk at a uniform pace and it may lift your spirits as well. There are several tapes on the market designed specifically to provide carefully selected walking music ranging from classical to calypso and including marches, light rock, country, and Latin rhythms. Speeds range from slow (105 steps a min) to brisk (up to 134 steps a min). Also, you can simply turn on the radio to a station you enjoy and walk away! You may find walking to music both energizing and relaxing and it can help the miles to fly by quickly. But be sure to keep the volume down low enough so that you can hear the noise of traffic and automobile horns. If you have to walk in the street, do not walk to music. You may prefer to savor the silence of a summer morning or a crisp winter afternoon, carrying with you only your own thoughts. The grand thing about walking is that you can do as you like.

FITNESS TRAIL

Combining a series of exercises with walking has become a very popular way to exercise. This concept originated in Switzerland with the "par cours" that was developed in the 1970s. The par cours (fitness trail) is a trail for walking or running, with exercise

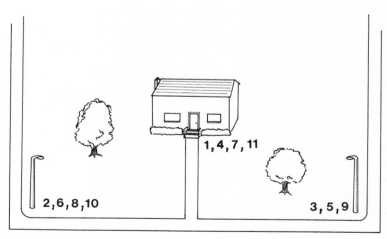

Figure 9.3. Fitness trail plan.

stations spaced along the way. It is now found in many city and town parks in this country as well. Figure 9.3 illustrates a typical course and outlines a sample plan of exercises to combine with walking. If there is no marked exercise route in your neighborhood, you can do the exercises using an existing park bench, armless straight-backed chair, a porch railing, or steps. You can walk out your front door, down to the corner and back, and do Exercise #1. Walk an equal amount of time or distance, and do Exercise #2, and so on. End by taking your pulse and then take a leisurely walk at a slower pace for a cool-down.

A Fitness Trail Outlined

Suggestions

1. This trail is designed so that exercises 1, 4, 7, and 11 are done by your front door; exercises 3, 5, and 9 are done at one end of the block or your turnaround point; and exercises 2, 6, 8, and 10 are done at the other end or turn-around point.
2. Some exercises require a "prop" such as a tree, a step or bench, a porch railing, or the door knob to assist you.

Station number	Exercise	Instructions	Repetitions	
			Beginner	Challenge
1	Head Turns and Tilts (#1, 2, pp. 100, 101) (Fig. 9.4)	Head is level. Turn to right and left. Tilt head to each side.	5 each side	10
2	Shoulder Shrugs (#9, p. 106) (Fig. 9.5)	Lift shoulders toward ears and then lower.	5	10
3	Arm Circles (#6, p. 104) (Fig. 9.6)	Circle straight arms forward. Circle straight arms back.	5	10

Station number	Exercise	Instructions	Repetitions	
			Beginner	Challenge
4	Push ups (#14, p. 110) (Fig. 9.7)	Standing, place hands on railing or tree; lower chest and push away. (Keep heels down.)	5	10
5	Leg Swings (#31, p. 124) (Fig. 9.8)	Stand by bench, tree, or railing and swing outside leg.	5 each leg	10
6	Twists or Side Bends (#5.8b, p. 92) (Fig. 9.9)	Sitting or standing, twist or bend to right and left.	5 each side	10
7	Forward Bend (Fig. 9.10)	Sitting, stretch arms up and slowly bend forward with chest between legs and arms extended.	5	10
8	Leg Lifts or Knee Lifts (Fig. 9.11)	Sitting or standing, lift straight leg or bring bent knee to chest. (If standing, hold on to a rail or tree.)	5 each leg	10
9	Demi-Pliés, Relevés (Fig. 9.12)	Stand behind a bench or by a tree with feet apart, heels down, back erect. Lower halfway and raise on toes.	5	10
10	Lower Leg Stretch (Fig. 9.13)	Stand behind bench or by a tree, one leg forward with knee bent, other leg back with knee straight. Lower heel to ground and hold.	2 each leg	4
11	Balance and Stretch (Fig. 9.14)	Stand on step or threshold by front door holding onto doorknob. Lower one heel at a time balancing on front part of foot on edge of step. Shift weight onto other leg and repeat.	2 each leg	4

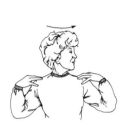 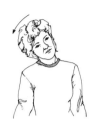 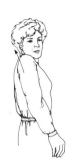

Figure 9.4. Neck turns and tilts.   Figure 9.5. Shoulder shrugs.

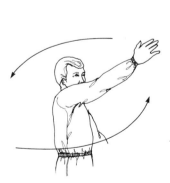 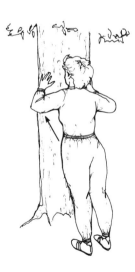

Figure 9.6. Arm circles.   Figure 9.7. Push-ups.

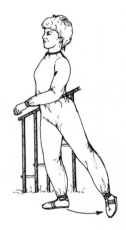

Figure 9.8. Leg swings.

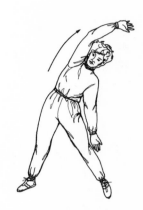

Figure 9.9. Twists or side bends.

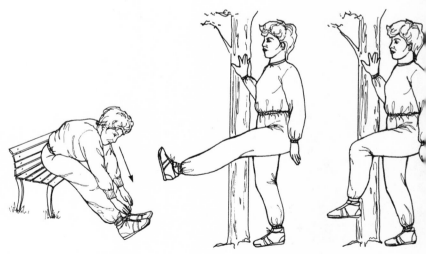

Figure 9.10. Forward bend.   Figure 9.11. Leg lifts or knee lifts.

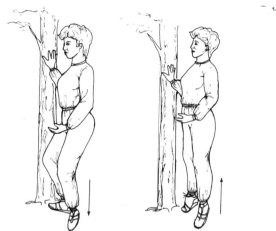

Figure 9.12. Demi-pliés and relevés.

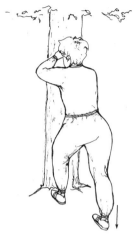

Figure 9.13. Lower leg stretch.

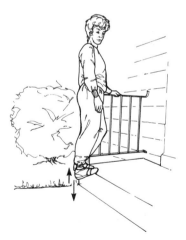

Figure 9.14. Balance and stretch.

KEEPING A RECORD

Staying motivated is not always easy. Ralph Waldo Emerson wrote that no one "is suddenly a good walker. Many men begin with good resolution, but they do not hold out." One way to keep up the good resolution to walk is to keep a record of your walking activities. Each time you walk, record the date, the time you spent walking, and your pulse rate at the start, halfway through, and at the end of your routine. Use the Record of Progressive Conditioning Program (Appendix J) to record your exercise progress. Look back at Table 5.1 for the suggested target heart rates for your age and at the 50% to 60% range. Also, monitor your rate of exertion. Keeping a record of this information will help you to see the progress you are making and motivate you to go on.

SUMMARY

Along with your walking program you may enjoy including another popular aerobic activity, cycling (discussed in the next chapter), to bring variety to your exercise program.

BIBLIOGRAPHY

References

Rippe, J.M., and Ward, A., 1989, *Rockport Walking Program*, New York, Prentice Hall.

Suggested Reading

Katsch, F. W., Wallace, J. P., VanCamp, S. P., and Verity, L., 1988, A longitudinal
    study of cardiovascular stability in active men aged 45 to 65 years, *Physician
    and Sportsmedicine* **16**(1):117–119, 122–123, 126.
Ralston, J., 1986, *Walking for the Health of It: The Easy and Effective Exercise for People
    Over 50*, Washington, D.C., Scott Foresman.
The Walking Magazine, published bi-monthly by Raben/The Walking Magazine
    Partners, 711 Boylston Street, Boston, MA 02116, Telephone: (617) 236-1885.

Resources

Keep Moving Program, Commonwealth of Massachusetts, Massachusetts, Execu-
    tive Office of Elder Affairs, 38 Chauncy St., Boston, MA 02111, Telephone: (617)
    727-4092.
National Organization of Mall Walkers, A.A.1 Box 60A, Hermann, MO 65041,
    Telephone: (314) 406-2601, attention: Tom Cabot.
Walker's Club of America (WCA), Boh M, Livingston Manor, NY 12750, Telephone:
    (914) 43999-5155, Howard Jacobson, President.
Walking Association, P.O. Box 37220, Tucson, AZ 85740, Telephone: (602) 742-9509.

CHAPTER 10
Cycling

I have two doctors—my left leg and my right leg.
Hindu Proverb

Using those two doctors to cycle is an excellent way to improve the aerobic capacity of your heart, lungs, and circulatory system. Cycling is an activity most people enjoy, and it can be done with little expense, in almost any community or neighborhood, or in your own home. Although cycling in a quiet neighborhood or park is a pleasant and relaxing way to exercise, in this chapter we will concentrate mainly on stationary bike cycling.

BASIC GUIDELINES

The following are some suggestions that will help you to select a bicycle and to get the most from your exercise on it.

1. The most important consideration is the height of the seat from the pedals. Adjust the bicycle seat so that when the foot is on the pedal the leg is almost but not quite straight.
2. A too-small bicycle seat can be very uncomfortable. It is possible to buy seats of various sizes that support the pelvis adequately, so "try them on" and choose the one that suits you best.
3. The use of toe straps helps keep the foot in place for the proper pedaling technique.
4. Warm-up stretches done before the beginning of a cycling session loosen the muscles and prevent injury or soreness. Concentrate on exercises that stretch the lower back, spinal muscles, quadriceps, gastrocnemius, and the muscles of the hip and hamstrings. The exercises in Table 10.1 are excellent for this. (See Chapter 6 for a complete description of the basic warm-up exercises.)
5. Cool-down stretches for the same body areas should be done after cycling. Do the exercises listed in Table 10.2

Table 10.1
Cycling Warm up

Exercise number	Exercise
1	Head Turns (p. 100)
2	Head Tilts (p. 101)
5	Single Arm Swings (p. 103)
6	Arm Circles (p. 104)
9	Shoulder Shrugs (p. 106)
13	Chest Stretch in Doorway (p. 109)
16	Pelvic Tilt (p. 112)
19	Knee-overs (p. 114)
31	Standing Leg Swings and Circles (p. 124)
33	Plié (p. 126)
34	Relevé (p. 127)
37	Prancing (p. 130)

Table 10.2
Cycling Cool down

Exercise number	Exercise
7	Wall Walk and Slide (p. 104)
13	Chest Stretch in Doorway (p. 109)
19	Knee-overs (p. 114)
30	Lower Leg Stretch at Wall (p. 123)
26	Cool-down Stretching (p. 120)
22	Pose of the Child (p. 116)

each time you finish your cycling session. (Again, see Chapter 6 for a full description of the exercises.) After the stretches, walk around the room or cycling space for about 2 to 5 min.

6. Record pulse, time, distance, and resistance setting on the bike (Table 10.3).

PRECAUTIONS

1. Breathe deeply while cycling to maintain the desired oxygen level.
2. Always monitor your pulse and your perceived rate of exertion, and record them.
3. Be aware that cycling can aggravate existing problems with knees.

EQUIPMENT

If you already own a bicycle, and if expense is a consideration, you may be interested to know that there are devices on the market that can temporarily convert your regular outdoor bike to a stationary bicycle. The cost is about $85.00 to $100.00. If you should decide to buy a new stationary bike, refer to the bike drawing as you fill in the checklist (Fig. 10.1).

Stationary bikes generally range in cost anywhere from $100.00 to $400.00. The deluxe-type Schwinn Air-Dyne cycle has handlebars that can also be adjusted for use as a rowing machine to give the upper body as well as the legs a conditioning workout. Various accessories can be purchased to enhance your enjoyment of stationary cycling. You can purchase an attachable book holder for about $10.00, and for those who prefer pleasant scenery while they exercise, there is even a videocassette tape (Cycle Vision) that provides a scenic bike trip right in your own living room. These are sold at many video and sporting goods stores.

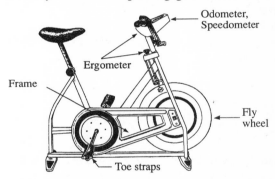

- Is the frame firm; does not wobble when you are pedaling? _____ Yes _____ No
- Is the fly wheel (the single wheel in the front) strong? _____ Yes _____ No
- Does the bike have toe straps? _____ Yes _____ No
- Is there an odometer that will measure the distance pedaled, or a speedometer to measure the miles per hour? _____ Yes _____ No
- Is there an ergometer to measure the amount of energy expended? _____ Yes _____ No
- Is there at least a 1-year warranty? _____ Yes _____ No
- Is repair service readily available? _____ Yes _____ No

Figure 10.1. Stationary bicycle checklist.

STATIONARY CYCLING PROGRAM

For those who are beginning a cycling program for the first time, the following plan is suggested:

1. Begin slowly in 5-min sessions, two times a day. Over 2 to 3 weeks, gradually increase the time to 12 min twice a day.
2. If no problems develop, increase the time to 20 min, once a day, cycling at a speed that puts your pulse rate within your appropriate target area. Do this at least 3 days a week.
3. Gradually build up to a total of 25 min a day. Always monitor your heart rate or your perceived rate of exertion. Increasing your speed and the resistance setting on the bicycle will give you a harder workout.
4. Record your information on Table 10.3 (see Appendix L).

ROAD CYCLING

This activity is more dangerous and is not recommended as a conditioning activity for the beginner. However, if you have been cycling safely all your life and are aware of the many safety considerations, there is no need for you to quit just because you have reached the age of 50, 60, or 70 years. But do wear a protective helmet and carry a clip-on water bottle on hot days. A red flag on a pole attached to the bicycle makes you much more visible to automobile drivers when you ride on busier roadways, as does bright, reflective clothing. Never listen to the radio or a tape while cycling on the open road. Check out the three-wheeled cycles too; they are a safe alternative and are gaining in popularity.

Table 10.3
Record of Cycling Conditioning Program

Date	Begin pulse[a]	Warm up	Halfway pulse[a]	Resistance	Distance/ Time Intensity	End pulse[a]	Cool down

[a]Count pulse for 6 sec, add a zero, and record.

SUMMARY

After exploring the variety of exercises that can be done in your own home, you may be ready for an activity that brings you together with others in a lively, sociable setting. If so, read the next chapter, which covers dancing.

BIBLIOGRAPHY

Suggested Readings

Ford, N., 1990, *Keep on Pedaling: The Complete Guide to Adult Bicycling*, Woodstock, Vermont, The Countryman Press.

Lawrence, R. M., and Rosenzweig, S., 1987, Exercise bicycles: Pedal power, in: *Going the Distance: The Right Way to Exercise for People Over 40*, Los Angeles, Jeremy Tarcher, Inc., pp. 89–97.

Mittleman, K., Crawford, S., Bhakthan, G., Guttman, G., and Holliday, S., 1986, Anthropometric changes in older cyclists: Effects of a trans-Canada bicycle tour, in: Day, J. A. P. (ed.), *Perspectives in Kinanthropometry*, Champaign, Illinois, Human Kinetics Publishers, pp. 107–113.

Chapter 11

Dancing as Exercise

On with the dance! Let joy be unconfin'd
Byron

Dancing can truly be a source of joy for the older adult, and it is wonderful exercise, too. Men and women have been enjoying various movement activities since the beginning of history, and things are not all that different today. It is a natural response for human beings to enjoy moving their bodies, and when movement is done to a definite rhythm or type of music, we call it "dancing." Dancing is a physical activity that is, first of all, great fun. In addition it offers an opportunity for social interaction and provides an excellent work-out. For many, it is the ideal form of exercise.

Dancing can be either structured (waltz, fox trot, polka) or it can be creative. It can be strenuous or done at a slow, comfortable pace. It can be done singly, with a partner, or as part of a line, square, or circle of others who also enjoy dancing. And though we have a definite idea of what dancing is all about, it is interesting to

213

know that it can even be done in a chair. This is especially meaningful for those who are weakened or disabled. So, dancing, in one form or another, can be done by nearly everyone. And dancing scores extremely high when it comes to meeting the physical, psychological, and social needs of older adults.

THE BENEFITS OF DANCING

The physical benefits of dance are numerous and include increased muscular strength and endurance, especially in the feet and legs; greater flexibility and increased joint mobility; improved circulation and aerobic capacity; and improved posture, balance, coordination, and grace.

Psychologically, the benefits include greater self-awareness and probably a better self-image. Negotiating the steps of a lively polka, a sedate line dance, or an intricate square dance routine does wonderful things for a person's self-image. It gives a real sense of accomplishment to be able to perform the dances and remember the steps. Also, it gives the mind a chance to relax from the cares of daily living and become totally absorbed in the movement of the dance.

As a social activity, dancing ranks high when it comes to meeting social needs. Through dance older adults can pass enjoyable times with old friends and make many new ones. Although dancing transcends all cultures, it is also an excellent way to learn about and appreciate other cultures as well. Dance also provides a perfect avenue for creative expression. Best of all, dancing and other forms of movement can be enjoyed throughout life. As role models, consider Martha Graham, one of the pioneers in the modern dance movement who maintained her involvement in dance into her 90s. Or Don Ameche, who amazed and delighted movie-goers with his dancing in the 1985 movie, *Cocoon*. Dance and other movement activities have much to offer at any age. The pleasure people derive from dancing is ageless.

BASIC GUIDELINES

Although dancing has always been a natural form of physical expression, there are some basic things to remember to make your dancing more enjoyable.

1. Keep your back erect. An erect back improves your posture and makes you look better and, more importantly, it takes much of the strain off your lower back and legs.
2. A relaxed body will allow you to dance more freely and smoothly. Keep your shoulders down and relaxed.
3. Keep your chest lifted and your seat tucked under slightly. This also improves your posture and allows you to breathe more deeply and freely.
4. Dance at a pace that is comfortable and pleasant for you. You should be able to talk with a partner or fellow dancer while you are dancing.
5. Remember to keep one foot on the floor all the time. This will lower the risk of stress fractures and damage to the ligaments, cartilage, and tendons in the knees and ankles. Also limit or avoid jumping or jerky movements.
6. Be sure the surface of the dance floor has some shock-absorbing qualities. Try to avoid dancing on unpadded, concrete floors—wooden floors are the most desirable.
7. Wear shoes with soles that slide easily on the floor no matter what kind of dancing you do. Overly high heels are not a good idea. And if you dance in bare feet, avoid any movements that involve much impact, since the foot is not protected by the impact-absorbing qualities of a shoe.

8. To guard against becoming dizzy and losing your balance, do not have your head lower than your waist for more than 20 sec.

WHAT TO WEAR

Generally speaking you can wear what you like to go dancing, although the type of shoe you choose for specific types of dances is important, as is making sure that your clothing is comfortable.

Shoes

If you are doing folk, square, jazz, or social dancing, a shoe with a leather sole and a 1-in heel will allow your foot to pivot and slide easily. Straps or laces keep the shoe snugly on the foot and prevent it from slipping on the heels, which causes blisters.

For low-impact aerobic dance, choose a shoe with a thick rubber sole to protect the ball and sole of the foot and absorb the force. One that flexes easily at the ball of the foot is best. Look for a sturdy heel cup, which will keep the ankle from turning. (Refer to the shoe discussion and Fig. 4.5 in Chapter 4 for more information.)

Clothing

Clothing should be comfortable and allow for ease of movement. Unless the occasion is formal, dresses or skirts, slacks, sport shirts, and other day wear are appropriate for folk, social, or square dancing. Slacks, shorts, leotards, and tights are best for low-impact aerobic dance, and for jazz, tap, or creative dancing where floor work is a possibility.

TYPES OF DANCE

There is a type of dance to suit every person and every personality. Following is a brief description, together with some historical information, about some of the most popular types.

"Jarming" or Chair Dancing

Chair dancing can be enjoyed by those who are no longer able to dance on their feet. The term "Jarming," an expression developed by Dr. Joseph D. Wassersug a retired internist from Quincy, Massachusetts, means jogging with the arms. He describes the benefits of this activity in his book, *Jarm: How to Jog With Your Arms to Live Longer*. He believes this pleasant activity "may significantly improve your general well-being and mental outlook and may also promote longevity" (Wassersug, 1984). Any arm, leg, and trunk movement done sitting can be put to music.

Social Dancing

Social dancing, sometimes called ballroom dancing, is dancing done with one partner at a time. In its various forms it has been popular since the early 1600s and its popularity continues today.

When dancing with a partner, it is the custom for the person "leading" to face counterclockwise and to begin the steps on the left foot. The person dancing as the "follower" faces clockwise and begins the steps on the right foot. The traditional flow of dancers on the dance floor is always counterclockwise.

Some historical notes, the step pattern, and the suggested music-beats to a measure, for the most common and popular dances follow. These dance steps can also be used when you are doing your own low-impact aerobic dance routines.

Waltz
(3/4 time)

Originated in Italy in the 16th century as a round dance called volte. The name is derived from the German word walzen meaning "to revalue."
Step pattern: step, side, close
        Count: 1   2   3

Fox Trot
(4/4 time)

The original dance was performed by a man named Harry Fox in a 1913 Broadway musical. The step was modified for social dance and became the most popular dance of that era in the United States; it is still widely danced today.
Step pattern: slow,   S,   quick, Q,   S,   S,   Q, Q,
        Count: 1–2, 3–4,   1,   2, 3–4, 1–2, 3,   4

Lindy Hop
(4/4 time)
(Swing)

Named after Charles Lindbergh, this dance originated in 1927 in the United States. It is the first of the "jitterbug" type dances.
Step pattern: toe–heel step, T–H step, step, step
        Count: 1+,   2+,   3,   4

Tango
(4/4 time)

This dance originated in Argentina in 1910, and is based on an earlier folk dance called the "Apache." The word "Tango" means "to have, own, or keep."
Step pattern: slow, slow, quick, quick, slow
        Count: 1–2, 3–4,   1,   2,   3–4

Rhumba
(4/4 time)

The rhumba originated in Cuba in the 1930s. The music shows the influence of African and Spanish cultures. The style is slow and relaxed.
Step pattern: quick, quick, slow
        Count: 1,   2,   3–4

Cha-Cha   This step also originated in Cuba, in 1955. The
(4/4 time)   steps are precise, and the style is light and gay.
                     Step pattern: slow, slow, Cha-Cha-Cha
                          Count: 1,   2,   3, & 4

Samba   This dance was first done in Brazil in 1929. The
(2/4 time)   music combines African and Latin American
                     rhythms. The style is lively with a springy knee
                     action.
                     Step pattern: quick and quick
                          Count: 1,   2,   3

Polka   This dance was the innovation of a Czech girl,
(2/4 time)   Anna Chadimova, in the early 1800s. The word
                     is derived from the Czech term "pulka," which
                     means half; referring to the half-step used in the
                     dance.
                     Step pattern: and quick and quick
                          Count: &   1   &   2

An offshoot of social dance, social dance aerobics, has recently been developed by Phil Martin and Dr. Betty Rose Griffith,
Professors of Physical Education at California State University at
Long Beach. Their 100-min videotape uses ballroom dances such
as the Swing (Lindy Hop), Cha-Cha, Polka, Samba, and Viennese
Waltz, for an aerobic conditioning effect. The tape is available by
mail. (For information on ordering, see Resources at the end of this
chapter.)

Folk Dance

Ethnic dances from a variety of cultures, which survive today
are known as folk dances, but the term also applies to characteris-
tic national dances, line dances, and figure dances, such as the
American square dance. These dances are often done in costume

to lively folk tunes and are especially popular at weddings and
ethnic restaurants and clubs. Folk dancing is very lively and can
elevate the pulse. Therefore check your pulse often and take deep
breaths. Some examples of well-known folk dances follow. (Folk
dance instructions are from Gilbert, C.; 1974, *International Folk
Dance at a Glance*, Minneapolis, Minnesota, Burgess Publishing Co.)

Hora   Israeli circle dance
(2/4 time)   Music: Hava Nagella
                    This dance is done in a circle; there are no partners.
                        Your hands are on your neighbors' shoulders.
                        The circle moves to the right. Wait measures 1–4
                        or 8 counts before beginning the step pattern.
                    Measures:
                    1–4   Introduction: wait
                    5–8   1   2   1   2   1   2
                            side behind side hop side hop
                              R   L   R   R   L   L
                    Step pattern just keeps repeating for rest of dance.

Miserlou   American version of a Greek line dance
(4/4 time)   Music: Miserlou, Never on Sunday
                    This dance is a line dance in which there are no
                        partners. The hands are joined at shoulder level
                        with the elbows bent. All dancers begin with the
                        right foot.
                    Measures
                    1–2   Introduction: wait
                    3–4   A. Face forward doing a grapevine step
                            1   2   3   4   1   2   3   4
                            step   point   back side front swing
                              R   L(no   L   R   L   R(no
                                    weight)   weight)

5–6   B. Face left for these slow two-steps.

1	2	3	4	1	2	3	4
step	close	step		back	close	back	
R	L	R		L	R	L	

Schottische Music: Swedish Schottische or Swedish Varsovinne
(4/4 or 2/4 Dancers may start on either foot and move in any
time)   direction then start the next schottische step on
             the other foot.
             The dance may be done two-by-two or in a long
             line.

1	2	3	4	1	2	3	4
step	step	step	hop	step	step	step	hop
L	R	L	L	R	L	R	R

Continue on repeating this step pattern till the
dance ends.

Polka   Music: Pennsylvania Polka or Clarinet Polka
(2/4 time) Dancers may start on either foot and move in any
            direction, then start the next polka step on the
            other foot.

ah	1	and	2
hop	step	close	step
R	L	R	L

Country Western

From quick and lively to slow and sentimental, this style of
dancing is enjoyable and appropriate for the older dancer. Many of
the dances are line dances so there is no need for a partner, and
this allows anyone who so desires, to join in. These dances are
especially popular throughout the Southern and Southwestern
states but are gaining in popularity throughout the country. The

Cotton-Eyed Joe, Freeze, and Four Corners are popular examples of Country Western line or circle dances.

Cotton-Eyed Joe

The formation of the dancers for the Cotton-Eyed Joe is a straight line, with any number of dancers. Arms are around the waist of the dancer on either side. Dancers at the end of the line put their outside arms on their hips.

Easy Version

1. Kick right foot twice.
2. March in place or move slightly backward three steps (R,L,R).
3. Kick left foot twice.
4. March in place or move slightly backwards three steps (L,R,L).
5. Repeat the kicks right and left—doing four times in all.
6. Beginning on the right, do eight triple steps forward (R,L,R–L,R,L).
7. Repeat from Step 1 until the music ends.

Variations

1. The dancers on the end can turn under the raised arm of the dancer next to them on Step 6.
2. The dancers on the end can finish the turn facing backward, thus they can repeat Steps 3, 4, and 5 while traveling backward.
3. The end dancers can switch with each other on the eight triple steps (Step 6), with one dancer traveling in back of the set and the other moving in front of the set simultaneously.

Freeze

This dance can be done to music in a 4/4 time such as "Party Time," "Tulsa Time," or even a disco number such as "Beat It" by Michael Jackson.

1. Grapevine to the right—Step on right foot, step behind with left, step to side with right, and lift left foot up with foot flexed (cowboy style). 4 counts.
2. Grapevine to the left—Step on left foot, step behind with the right, step to the side with the left, and lift the right foot up with foot flexed (cowboy style). 4 counts.
3. Step back on right, left, right and lift left foot. 4 counts.
4. Step forward on the left foot—2 counts; and back on the right foot—2 counts, doing the "rock step."
5. Step on the left foot as you turn to face to the left and hold up right foot. 4 counts.
6. Dance is now repeated facing this direction and you continue this way until the music ends.

Four Corners

This dance is also done to music in 4/4 time. Popular songs for this dance are "Elvira," "Bobbie Sue," and "Swinging."

1. Begin with the feet together and twist the heels to the left, then right, and repeat 3 more times. 8 counts.
2. Touch right heel forward, touch right toe beside left foot, and touch right heel forward, and step right. 4 counts.
3. Touch left heel forward, touch left toe back (no weight on it), step forward with left and lift up right knee, and step in place with right foot. 4 counts.
4. Touch left toe back for 4 counts.
5. Step forward on left, raise right knee, step on right and touch left toe beside right foot. 4 counts. Repeat 3 times

and, as the right knee is up the last time, turn to face left (Say to yourself "Step, lift, step, touch 3 times" and the fourth time say "Step, and turn").

6. Now do grapevine step moving toward the left but beginning with the right foot stepping in front of left, left foot steps to side left, and then right foot steps behind left. 3 counts.

7. Weight is on the right foot as you touch left to side and step on it 2 counts, and touch the right foot to the side and step bringing feet together 2 counts.

8. Dance begins again with the swivel steps in Step 1 and is repeated as you turn to face a new direction, eventually forming a square pattern on the floor.

Line Dances

Line dances are very popular because a partner is not required. The music is usually a familiar popular song. The movement patterns are usually simple but can always be made more complicated. Arm movements can be added as well. There is also the opportunity for dancers to add their own little variations such as hip wiggles and shoulder shrugs. The directions for several popular line dances follow.

The Birdie Dance

This dance is very funny because you mimic the antics of a bird. You begin by standing with your arms at your sides in a circle, line, or facing another person if you wish. There is a wait for eleven counts at the introduction and you have to be ready to begin the "birdie " movements on the upbeat of count 12. There are two basic parts which are designated as Part A and Part B.

Part A

1. Raise your arms with your hands in front of you palms facing away. Make a "beak" with your fingers and do 4 quack-like movements with the thumb and fingers. 4 counts.
2. Flap your arms 4 times like a bird with the elbows out and forearms facing inward and fingers in armpits. 4 counts.
3. Bend your knees slightly and wiggle your hips 4 times. 4 counts.
4. Clap your hands 4 times. 4 counts.

Part B

There are several ways you can do this part. The feet can be doing a simple walking step to the music or you can be doing a two-step, or a Polka step.

1. If you are in a circle you can all join hands and do the steps 8 counterclockwise and then 8 clockwise.
2. Or you can link arms with one other person and do the steps.
3. Or you can make a right-hand star with another person and turn twice around, and change and make a left-hand star for 8 steps.
4. Music will cue you when to begin Part A.

You continue the dance by repeating Parts A and B until the song ends.

Hallelujah

This is a simple line dance done to the song "Hallelujah" by Parker and Penny. The words to the song are beautiful and lend themselves easily to group singing. This dance can also be adapted for "Chair Dancing."

1. Standing with arms overhead sway to the left, right, left, and right. 4 counts.
2. Walk sideways to the right starting on the left foot: left, right, left, right. 4 counts.
3. Sway again left, right, left, right. 4 counts.
4. Walk sideways to the left starting on the left foot: left, right, left, right. 4 counts.
5. Walk forward left, right, left and touch right heel forward. 4 counts (You can lean back and raise hands up in praise attitude if you want).
6. Walk backward right, left, right; touch left toe back. 4 counts.
7. Walk forward left, right and cross left in front of right, step back on right. 4 counts.
8. Repeat Step 7. 4 counts.
9. Repeat dance in its entirety until song ends.

Sweet Georgia Brown

This is a fun dance that can be done to the song by this name but the step pattern can be done to most 4/4 time music that is "jazzy." This is a dance that can be done with people scattered around the dance floor. It works best though when everyone begins by facing the same direction, which we will designate as front.

1. Turn left and walk 4 steps. 4 counts.
2. Walk 4 steps back. 4 counts.
3. Moving to the right, do the 8-step grapevine. 8 counts. (This is done by stepping to the right on the right foot, step behind with the left foot, side with the right foot and across front with the left foot, step to the side with the right, behind with the left, to the side with the right, and across front with the left.)

4. With the weight on the left foot, turn to the left doing 4 Buzz Steps. (This is done by turning left foot out to side slightly and taking the weight on the foot, and stepping on the right foot to allow the left foot to pivot you around until you are back facing the direction in which you started the 4 Buzz Steps.) 4 counts.

5. Turning to the right, do 4 Buzz Steps (step and pivot). 4 counts.

6. Do 2 steps to the left and 2 steps to the right and repeat. Total 8 counts.

7. Repeat the entire dance.

12th Street Rag

This step pattern will fit with other Ragtime music but is especially fun to do with the song by this name. Again the time is 4/4.

1. Weight is on the right foot and you begin the step with the left toe touching forward, left toe touching side and then step in place left, right, left. 8 counts.

2. Repeat the above pattern with the right foot. 8 counts.

3. Do 4 "Limp steps" to the left. 8 counts. Limp steps are done by stepping to the left with the left foot and dragging the right foot over beside the left and doing 3 more.

4. Now do 4 "Limp steps" to the right. 8 counts.

5. Do 2 Charleston steps. 8 counts. This step is done by stepping to the left with the left foot and touching right toe forward and then back and stepping on to the right and touching left toe behind. (Say to yourself "Step, touch forward, step, touch back.")

6. You are now ready to repeat the step pattern until the music ends.

Low-Impact Aerobic Dance

Take it easy here and choose an aerobics program in which only movements that do not jar the body are done. The best are low-impact aerobics (LIA) or non-impact aerobics (NIA). In these dance moves, one foot is kept in contact with the floor at all times, there is no jumping or running, and the movements are smooth and slow rather than fast or jerky. The music should follow a comfortable tempo and you should be able to move to it easily. If the tempo is slow, do one movement with each beat; if the tempo is faster, do one movement to every two or even four beats.

You can easily create your own low-impact dance routine by simply combining a few basic movements, beginning with a walk, then changing directions forward, backward, and diagonally. Stepping to the side with one foot crossing in front or crossing behind then becomes a grapevine step. Low kicks can also be added, as can arm movements in all directions. Finally, claps and finger snaps can be included to create a lively, upbeat feeling. Turn on the radio to a station whose music you like. Then just do any movements you enjoy, adding some movements to stretch the muscles of the torso. Continue for up to 15–20 min, slowing down when you need to. Remember, you can always incorporate some social dance and folk dance step patterns or steps from the various line dances. This is an especially creative way to enjoy dancing and it is also a great deal of fun.

Ballet

Many people appreciate the more disciplined and structured approach of ballet as a form of dance and exercise. Ballet exercises done at a ballet barre, counter, or by the back of a chair are an excellent way to increase the muscle strength of the legs and abdomen and to improve posture. Keep in mind the following guidelines, whether standing at a barre, a counter, or a chair.

1. Do the exercises either barefoot or wearing ballet slippers.
2. Hold the spine erect. Do not sink.
3. When standing, always hold the muscles at the front of the thigh (quadriceps) firm; this lifts the knee caps and keeps the gluteal muscles of the seat tight.
4. Contract the abdominal muscles and feel the lift from the inside of the body. Hold, release, and repeat.
5. Hold your head up and balanced on the spine, with a feeling of lightness.

See Fig. 11.1 for the incorrect alignment and Fig. 11.2 for the correct alignment emphasized in the guidelines 1–4.

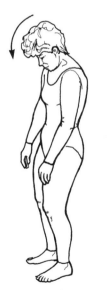
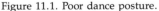
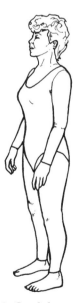

Figure 11.1. Poor dance posture.   Figure 11.2. Good dance posture.

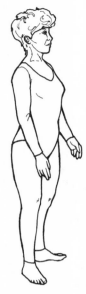

Figure 11.3. Ballet: first position.

The following exercises are suitable for you to do at home. As you do them, be aware of your body, the muscles you are using, and the feelings you are experiencing. Play a record or tape of some classical or semiclassical music you enjoy while doing these exercises.

1. **Prancing**; #37, Fig. 6.37 (p. 130).
2. **Posture:** Lift the head and press the shoulders down.
3. **First Position** (Fig. 11.3).
   a. Heels are together and the arch of the foot is lifted. The weight of the body is over the balls of the feet.
   b. The spine is positioned slightly forward with the torso lifting up and out of the hips.

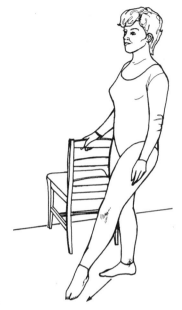

Figure 11.4. Battements tendus, to the front.

    c. Weight is balanced equally on each foot.

    d. Contract the abdominal muscles, as described in Guideline 4. Hold, release, and repeat.

4. **Demi-Plié**; Fig. 6.33 (p. 126): Do 8.

5. **Relevé**; Fig. 6.34 (p. 127): Do 8.

6. **Battements Tendus to the Front** (Fig. 11.4): Do 8 with each leg.

    a. Keep both legs turned out at all times, knees pointed to the sides.

    b. Slide the heel forward until the foot is stretched, with toes slightly touching the floor. Now lift the heel and hold for 2 counts.

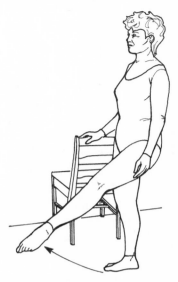

Figure 11.5. Battements tendus, to the front.

c. Lift the leg to the front and keep the toes pointed. Think about lifting the torso out of the supporting leg. Hold for 2 counts (Fig. 11.5).

    d. Lower the leg, using the muscles of the back.

    e. Slide the foot back to the original position without letting the knees bend. Hold for 2 counts.

7. **Battements Tendus to the Side**. Do 8 with each leg.

    a. Point the center of the knee toward the ceiling, keep the foot fully pointed, and slide the foot to the side. Hold for 2 counts (Fig. 11.6).

    b. Lift the leg, keeping both thighs turned out. Hold for 2 counts (Fig. 11.7).

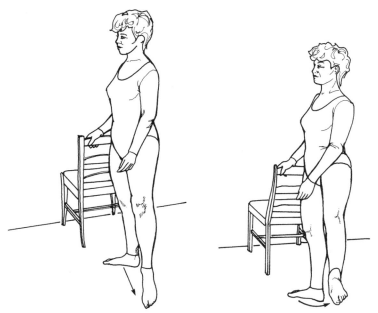

Figure 11.6. Battements tendus, to the side.

Figure 11.7. Battements tendus, to the side.

  c. Lower the leg to the floor with the foot still pointed. Hold for 2 counts.
  d. Slide the foot back to the original position. Hold for 2 counts.

SUMMARY

Having read and tried some of these approaches to dance, you most probably have experienced the joy that can come from dancing. This joy and freedom of movement can also be experi-

enced when doing aquatic activities, which will be discussed in
the following chapter.

BIBLIOGRAPHY

References

Berryman-Miller, S., 1988, Dance/movement: Effects on elderly self-concept, *Journal of Physical Education, Recreation and Dance* **59**(5):42–46.

Caplow-Lindner, E., Harpaz, L., Samberg, S., 1979, *Therapeutic Dance/Movement* New York, Human Sciences Press.

Corbin, D. E., and Metal-Corbin, J., 1990, *Reach For It*, 2nd ed., Dubuque, IA, Eddie Bowers Publishing Company.

Rogers, C. C., 1986, Upper body exercise: "Jarming" instead of jogging, *The Journal of The Physician and Sports Medicine* **14**(5):181–186.

Rosas, D., Rosas, C., and Martin, K., 1987, *Non-Impact Aerobics*, New York, Hard Books.

Wassersug, J. D., 1984, *Jarm: How to Jog with Your Arms to Live Longer*, Port Washington, NY, Ashley Books, Inc.

Welles, L., 1982, *Ballet Body Book*, Indianapolis, The Bobbs-Merrill Company, Inc.

Videotapes

Social Dance Aerobics, Prime Time Aerobics, Suite 130, 3089 C, Clairemont Drive, San Diego, CA 92111.

Arm Chair Fitness, C.C.-M. Productions, 7755 16th Street, N.W., Washington, D.C. 20012.

Dancin' Grannies Exercise Program, 1989 Dancin' Grannies, Suite #3, 10 Bay Street, Westport, CT 06880.

Records

Lindnor, E. C., and Harpaz, L., *Special Dancing on Your Feet or in Your Seat*, Educational Activities, Inc., Freeport, NY 11520.

Lindnor, E.C., Samberg, S., and Harpaz, L., *Special Music for Special People*, Education Activities, Inc., Freeport, NY 11520.

CHAPTER 12

Aquatic Activities

To be active is the primary vocation of man
Goethe

Water activities, both swimming and nonswimming, are becoming increasingly popular forms of exercise. More and more people are enjoying the satisfying and relaxing benefits of being in the water, the way it helps relieve their tensions and worries, and the new feelings of confidence and self-worth it imparts. Older swimmers, particularly those who have some difficulty getting around, appreciate the wonderful freedom of movement that being in the water provides.

In this chapter we will discuss in detail the benefits of exercising in the water, as well as reviewing some precautionary measures. Instructions for suitable exercises and sample workouts are also included. No swimming skill is necessary to do the aquatic exercises. If you choose to do the fitness swimming using swimming strokes, just follow the sample workouts. For instructions on perfecting your swimming strokes you might want to read *Swimming For Seniors* by Ed Shea. This is an excellent book for helping the older adult to use swimming as a conditioning program. Swimming is strongly recommended as a means of exercise because it provides the participant with improved muscular strength, endurance, and flexibility, as well as improved respiratory and cardiovascular fitness. Most important, all of this is accomplished safely and without the compression of joints that can occur when exercising on land. Many call it the perfect form of exercise.

BENEFITS

Although exercising in the water provides an excellent workout for people of all ages, the following unique qualities make it especially beneficial for the older exerciser.

1. Your body becomes more buoyant in water, where it weighs only 10% of its actual weight; thus, a 150-lb person weighs only 15 lbs in the water when submerged to the neck. Because of this, you can move more easily and more comfortably in the water.
2. The water's buoyancy acts as a cushion for your body, allowing it to float and giving the joints greater freedom from the effects of gravity. There is less trauma when doing an exercise in the water compared to that for the same exercise done out of the water.
3. The water also provides resistance for the muscles as you move your body through it. This improves muscular strength.
4. This water resistance also creates an aerobic conditioning effect on the heart and lungs.

PRECAUTIONS

Water activities are among the safest of all the sports and exercise activities. Nevertheless, you should keep in mind a few simple precautions when you are exercising in the water.

1. Do your water exercises with a friend or when a lifeguard is present.
2. Enter the pool by the stairs or steps, holding onto the handrail (Fig. 12.1). If it is a ladder-style step, turn around and face the side of the pool with your back to the water and carefully lower yourself, finding each step with your foot before you transfer your weight onto that step.
3. Perform the movements through as full a range of motion as is comfortable. Do not overdo the leg movements, because these can overstrain and aggravate the lower back.

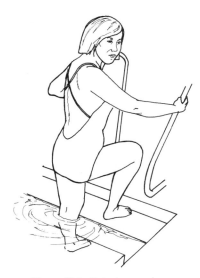

Figure 12.1. Entering pool.

4. If you have a balance problem, position yourself near the pool edge for standing exercises.

5. Make sure that the water temperature is at a comfortable level (84–86°F).

GUIDELINES

Here are a few practical guidelines to help you get the most benefit from your water exercise program.

1. Always shower with soap before and after your session in the pool.

2. If you have been a nonswimmer all of your life, position yourself in chest-high water near the side of the pool until you feel more at ease in the water and gain confidence.

3. If you have a hearing or vision problem, position yourself near the instructor, if there is one, or near another person who is following the exercise directions, so that it is easier for you to participate. If you wear glasses, you may keep them on in the pool, since the exercises are done with the head above the water. An elastic headband to keep them in place can be helpful as well. For swimming you may want to wear ear plugs and also swim goggles.

4. Many women prefer to wear swim caps, but when they are pulled down they greatly muffle any exercise instructions that may be given. You can fold the cap up above the ears to hear better, or wear a shower cap to protect your hair.

5. Some people are ill-at-ease wearing a swim suit, but the benefits gained from exercising will help a great deal in overcoming this feeling, if only the water program is given a chance. You may also wear shorts and a T-shirt if you wish.

6. Always monitor your pulse, especially after doing a series of walking, skipping, or leg exercises, or after continuous swimming.
7. Always take a drink before and after your exercise session in the water.
8. Take many deep breaths during the exercising.
9. If you have difficulty staying afloat in a horizontal position, there are belts and vests to assist you. Also, if you want to "run" in deep water, there is a vest that keeps you in a vertical position.

AQUATIC EXERCISES

A variety of programs of aquatic exercise have been developed as an outgrowth of physical therapy and hydrotherapy programs. The Arthritis Foundation is encouraging participation in water exercises, and in some states sponsors a training program for instructors, called Aqua Joints. To locate an Aqua Joints class in your area, contact your local pool or the Arthritis Foundation (Resources section).

The following is a program of beginner- and challenge-level water exercises. Each is about 25–30 min in length.

Beginner Level

Warm up

1. **Walk** continuously in chest-deep water for 3–4 min.
2. **Toe Raises**: Rise up on toes 15 times.
3. **Side Bender**: Stand with legs apart and gently lean to each side, letting the arm reach over your head to increase the stretch. Do 10 on each side.

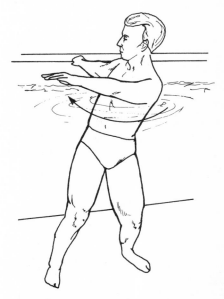

Figure 12.2. Trunk twists.

4. **Trunk Twists** (Fig. 12.2): Stand with legs apart, knees slightly bent, arms shoulder-high. Gently move arms from side to side, allowing your back to turn to stretch gently. Do 16 times.

5. **Front and Back Clapping**: Move arms in the water to clap; 10 times in the front and 10 times in the back.

6. By the pool wall, do the following:
   Leg Swings: Forward and back 10 times. Swing the leg that is toward the center of the pool.
   Leg Circles: Circle forward 10 times, and then reverse and do 10 more. Turn around and repeat both exercises with the other leg.

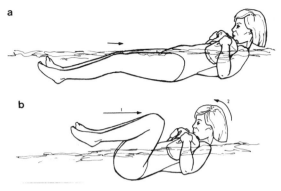

Figure 12.3. Sit-up.

Aerobic Workout

1. **Sit-ups**: Use two plastic milk or water jugs (1-gal size) as flotation devices. Hold them under the arms, and while floating, bring the knees to the chest and then extend them back out, remaining on your back (Fig. 12.3a). Now, bring the knees to the chest, and while you are in a tuck position (Fig. 12.3b), slowly lean forward and extend the legs out straight behind you (Fig. 12.4). You are now on your front. Bring the knees to the chest and gently return to your back. Repeat this motion, working your abdominal muscles. Breathe normally. Do 10 with the legs forward and 10 with the legs back.

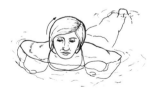

Figure 12.4. Sit-up.

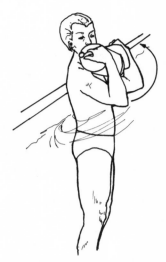

Figure 12.5. Biceps curls.

2. **Biceps Curls**: Now fill the jugs with 1, 2, or 3 in of water to make them heavier. They will now serve as "weights." Holding your arms out in front of you, bend your elbows, bringing the jugs to touch your shoulders (Fig. 12.5). Breathe normally. Do 10 times. (If the jugs feel too heavy, pour out some water.)
3. **Triceps Firmer**: Stand erect, holding the jugs, and raise one arm at a time over your head, keeping your bent elbow next to your ear. Then straighten your arm using the muscle of the back of the upper arm, the triceps, to do this motion (Fig. 12.6). Breathe normally. Repeat with the other arm. Do 10 with each arm.
4. **Chest and Shoulders Strengthener**: Stand erect. Holding your arms out in front of you, move the jugs forward and backward in the water. Do 10 in each direction.
5. **Leg Kicks**: Empty the water from the jugs and hold them under your arms to assist you in floating. Now, do a kick

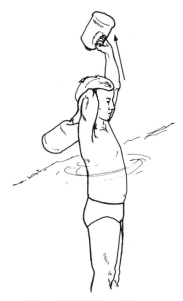

Figure 12.6. Triceps firmer.

stroke with the legs propelling you through the water, either on your back or on your stomach, for 2–3 min (Fig. 12.7). If you are a novice in the water you may wish to do the kick while holding on to the side of the pool. You may do any kick you want, changing if you feel like it from a flutter to a frog kick. These leg kicks are what will start to elevate the pulse, so take your pulse now.

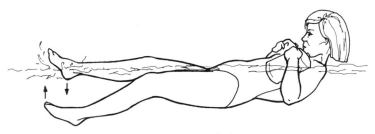

Figure 12.7. Leg kicks.

6. **Marching**: Set the empty jugs on the side of the pool. Now do a march in the water, with stiff arms and legs, for 2–3 min.

7. **Bent Knee Trunk Twists**: Position yourself by the pool wall. Floating on your back and holding onto the pool side, bring the knees in toward the chest and then take the bent knees over to the side. Move back to the center and over to the other side (Fig. 12.8). Do 10 to each side.

8. **Bent Knee to Opposite Shoulder**: Standing with your back to the side of the pool and holding on to the side, bend the right knee and bring it toward the left shoulder (Fig. 12.9). Repeat with the left knee. Do 10 with each leg.

Cool down

1. **Side Leans**: Hold onto the pool side with the right hand and place the feet one in front of the other where the pool floor and wall meet. Then extend the right arm, allowing the body to move out toward the center of the pool, and bring the left arm up over the head for a nice stretch (Fig. 12.10). Hold and enjoy it, and then repeat on the other side.

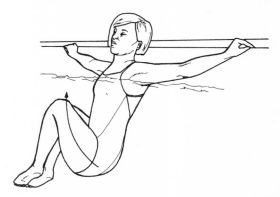

Figure 12.8. Bent knee trunk twist.

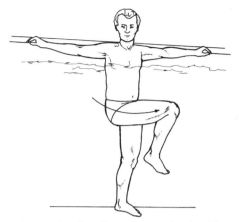

Figure 12.9. Bent knee to opposite shoulder.

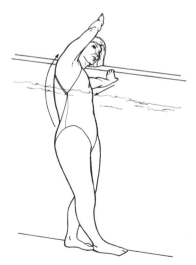

Figure 12.10. Side leans.

2. **Pelvic Circles**: Stand with the feet wider than your hips, knees bent, and hands on hips. Now move the pelvis forward, then to the right, then to the back, over to the left, and then forward. Make this a smooth, continuous, circular movement. Do 5 clockwise, then reverse and do 5 more counterclockwise.

3. **Side Lunges**: Face the pool wall and hold on with the hands. Stand with the legs wide apart and lower yourself to each side, bending the knees and allowing the muscles of the inner thigh to stretch gently (Fig. 12.11). Do 5 to each side.

4. **Wall Climb**: Face the wall, standing an arm's length away and holding onto the side with both hands. Start to walk the legs up the wall, trying to keep them straight to gently stretch the hamstrings at the back of the thigh (Fig. 12.12). When you get the feet as high as you comfortably can, gently sway from side to side enjoying the gentle stretch in the back and ribs.

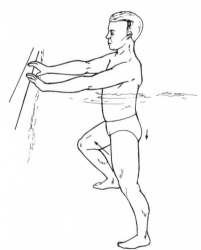

Figure 12.11. Side lunges.

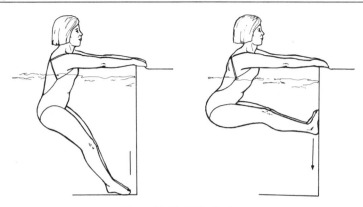

Figure 12.12. Wall climb.

5. **Ship's Figurehead**: Stand with your back to the pool wall and hold on with your hands. Keeping the heels touching the wall, allow yourself to gently lean forward like a ship's figurehead (Fig. 12.13).

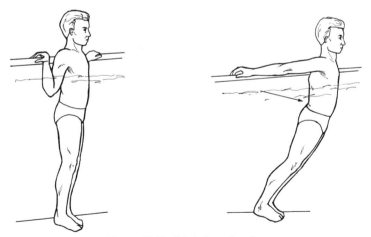

Figure 12.13. Ship's figurehead.

Challenge Level

Warm up

1. **Walk** continuously in chest-deep water doing **Arm Circles** for 3–4 min.
2. **Ankle Circles**: Standing on left leg do ankle circles with right ankle, do a foot flex and then point the toe. Do the same with the left ankle and foot. Do 6–8 to each side.
3. **Prance** over to the wall, raising knees and pointing toes.
4. **Leg Swings**: At the pool side do 10 leg swings with each leg.
5. **Flamingo**: Standing with your back to the wall, bring a bent leg up and then out to the side (Fig. 12.14). Repeat with the other leg. Do this for 1–1½ min.
6. **Hip Dip**: Stand with your side to the wall and the arm that is holding onto the pool side straight. Keep the feet flat,

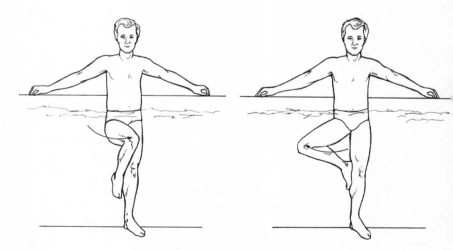

Figure 12.14. Flamingo.

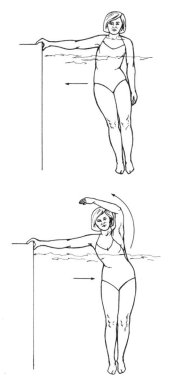

Figure 12.15. Hip dip.

and then push the hip toward the wall and away (Fig. 12.15). Do 10 and then change and do 10 with the other hip.

7. **Hula Hoop**: Stand with your back to the wall and move the hips in a full circle. Reverse and do for 1 min.

8. **Bent Knee to Opposite Shoulder**: Stand with back to the wall, arms holding the sides of the pool. Bring the right knee up toward the left shoulder. Repeat with the left knee to the right shoulder (Fig. 12.9). Do 6–8 with each leg.

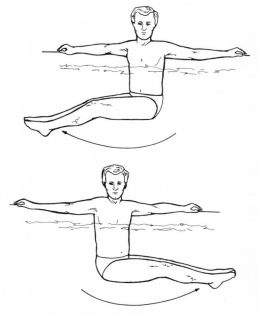

Figure 12.16. Windshield wipers.

9. **Windshield Wipers with Legs**: If you have problems with
   your lower back, don't do this one. Standing with your
   back to the pool, hands holding on the the pool edge, bring
   up both legs and swing them to the right and then to the
   left (Fig. 12.16). This is not easy. Try to keep your back
   pressed into the pool wall using the abdominal muscles to
   assist you.

Aerobic Workout

It's fun to do these exercises to lively music.

1. **Skip**: for 1 or 2 min.
2. For 1–2 min, do three steps and then a kick. If you are doing this with a class or with friends, it is fun to hold on to the waist of the person in front of you to form a "Conga Line."
3. **Step and kick** continuously across the width of the pool. If you are doing this with friends or as part of a class, stand side-by-side with arms around each other's waists and form a "Chorus Line." Take your pulse.
4. **Water Dance**: (This can be done by yourself or with a partner.) Do three stride jumps and clap twice. (Stride jumps are done by jumping with legs apart and then together. Legs can go either to the side or one forward and one back in an alternating pattern.) Repeat this pattern 3 times. Then, moving in a circle to your right, take 8 steps and reverse, moving in a circle to your left. If you have a partner, do Elbow Swings with the right elbows hooked for 8 steps, and then to the left with left elbows joined. Then repeat, doing four stride jump-claps followed by Elbow Swings. Take your pulse.
5. If you need further aerobic activity, do some leg kicks, on either your back or front, using kickboards or plastic jugs to assist you in floating; or do them by the side of the pool. Take your pulse.

Cool down

1. **Leg Swings** by the side of the pool.
2. **Calf Stretch**: Stand facing the pool with forearms resting

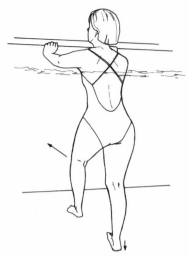

Figure 12.17. Calf stretch.

on the pool gutter. The left foot is forward with the knee bent, and the right foot is back with the heel on the pool floor and the leg straight, to stretch gently. Hold and then switch legs so the right leg is forward and the left leg is back (Fig. 12.17).

3. **Wall Climb**: described in Step 4 of the beginner-level cool-down (Fig. 12.12).
4. **Ship's Figurehead**: described in Step 5 of the beginner-level cool-down (Fig. 12.13).

FITNESS SWIMMING PROGRAM

For those older adults who know how to swim, we strongly recommend that you pursue swimming as a nearly ideal exercise program. As mentioned previously, the benefits to the total body are great. Speed is not important, but it is suggested that any strokes may be combined for a 20- to 30-min continuous swim at least three days a week. The pulse can be monitored to keep at the desired target heart rate level, but also watch for all of the warning signs of overexertion that are discussed in Chapter 5. If you are experiencing muscular weakness, aches and pains, or persistent tiredness during the day, you are probably overdoing and should try the following suggestions: (1) slow down your swimming pace, (2) have a rest period during your swimming time, or (3) stop swimming that day.

You should always record your exercise routine (Table 12.1 and Appendix M). Most pools are 25 yards (or 25 meters) long. You can record the distance you swim in laps or partial laps (a lap is two lengths), or in yards. Record, too, the date, the distance you swam continuously without stopping to rest, how much time you swam continuously, and your total workout time. Also write down any comments on how you felt, what strokes you used, and your pulse rate when you completed your continuous swim or halfway through your workout.

Beginner- and challenge-level fitness swimming programs follow.

Beginner Level (25–100 yards)

Warm up

1. Do the warm-up exercises described in the aquatic exercise section for 5 min.
2. Do stroke practice for 5 min.

Table 12.1
Record of Aquatics Conditioning Program

Date	Begin pulse[a]	Warm up	Pulse[a]	Exercise or swim	Distance/ time intensity	Exercise pulse[a]	Cool down

[a]Count pulse for 6 sec, add a zero, and record.

Aerobic Workout

Begin by swimming one pool length, and gradually add 25 yards to your total distance until you can swim that distance continuously. Then keep increasing your distance each time you swim until you are able to swim 100 yards, or four pool lengths, continuously. Take your pulse and monitor your body's response.

Cool down

1. Swim at a slower pace using a resting stroke, such as the breast stroke or side stroke, or walk around in the shallow end for 5 min or until your pulse has slowed.
2. Do the cool-down stretches that are listed in the aquatic exercise section.

Challenge Level (100–300 yards)

Warm up

1. Do the warm-up exercises described in the aquatic exercise section for 5 min.
2. Do stroke practice for 5 min.

Aerobic Workout

Swim 100 yards and then, without stopping, attempt to swim further, trying for 10 to 20 more feet. Take your pulse.

Rest and then do a cool-down swim. Swim 50 yards and then rest again. You can repeat this cool-down swim, with a rest period, two or three more times depending on how you feel. Do not overdo it.

Cool down

1. Walk in the shallow end for awhile.
2. Do the cool-down stretches that are listed in the aquatics exercise section.

SUMMARY

If you have been a swimmer, you will probably enjoy getting back into the water. If you have not been a swimmer or spent much time in the water, try it now. You will be amazed at how relaxing and enjoyable aquatic activities can be.

As Goethe said, being active should be our primary vocation. Since you are becoming more active or are remaining active then you will most probably be interested in the information in Chapter 13. You may want to try some activities that will allow you to stretch and grow, and even to challenge your competitive spirit. The extras that follow may open new doors for you.

BIBLIOGRAPHY

References

De Varona, D., and Tarshis, B., 1984, *Donna DeVarona's Hydro-Aerobics*, New York, Macmillan.

Katz, J., 1985, *The Water Exercise Technique Workout*, New York, Facts on File Publications.

Shea, E. J., 1986, *Swimming for Seniors*, Champaign, Illinois, Leisure Press.

Suggested Readings

Ekberg, J., 1990, Senior fitness: Getting into the swim of things, *Parks and Recreation* **25**(2):46–49.

Evenbeck, B., 1986, Aquatic exercise—taking shape, *Journal of Physical Education, Recreation, and Dance* **57**(10):22–25.

Giles, M., 1988, *Aquacizes: Restoring and Maintaining Mobility with Water Exercise*, Bedford, Mass., Mills and Sanderson.

Lee, T., 1984, *Aquacises: Terry Lee's Waterworkout Book*, Englewood Cliffs, NJ, Prentice-Hall.

McWaters, J. G., 1988, *Deep Water Exercise for Health and Fitness*, Laguna Beach, Calif., Publitec Publishing.

Perry, P., 1986, Weightless workouts, *American Health—Fitness of Body and Mind* **5**(5):78–81.

Resources

Swim America, American Swim Coaches Association, 1 Hall of Fame Drive, Fort Lauderdale, FL 33316, Telephone: (305)462-6267.

CHAPTER 13

Something Extra

Life is so rich and full these days.
There is so much to look forward to, so much
here and now, and also ahead.
At Seventy, May Sarton

Throughout our lives there are new ideas to be explored, new challenges to be faced and met, and new goals to be reached. All of us know vigorous, intelligent older people who, well into their 70s and beyond, are still learning and growing. In the area of exercise, there are many opportunities for the older adult to broaden his or her exercise experience and to meet some challenges, if desired. All of the activities described in this chapter provide the extra enrichment that many seniors seek.

ELDERHOSTEL

Elderhostel is composed of programs of enrichment, held on university campuses, that many times offer exercise. Attendance at Elderhostels has increased dramatically since the first ones were organized in 1975 by Marty Knowlton with 200 participants at five New Hampshire campuses. In 1990, more than 190,000 participants were registered in Elderhostel programs in the United States. Over fifty foreign countries also hosted Elderhostel programs.

Those attending the programs usually live in the college dormitories (usually for one week), eat in the dining hall, take courses taught by college faculty members, enjoy the use of the libraries and campus facilities, and attend special events. There are no education requirements, but participants and their companions must be 60 years of age or older. There are three basic rules that participating colleges or universities must follow: (1) the basic fee is set by the Elderhostel Board of Directors and cannot exceed that total cost for the week; (2) the courses must be taught by regular faculty members at a level equal to the regular academic program; and (3) none of the courses may teach the hosteler "How to Grow Old."

When choosing an Elderhostel site and program look for one that also offers a class in exercise. For example, Hatha Yoga, Healthy Heart Exercise, Swimnastics, and Dance have been offered at Ball State University, Muncie, Indiana, since the program began in 1979. The exercise class is taught by a knowledgeable, trained physical education professional from among the regular faculty. For more information, see the Resources section.

SENIOR OLYMPICS

For those who are in good health, enjoy athletic competition, and are actively involved in a program of physical conditioning, the Senior Olympics, or Senior Games as they are sometimes called, provide an opportunity to compete against others of the same age and sex in a great many sports and activities. These Games are closely modeled after the Olympics, with some modifications to the rules and equipment. The first United States National Senior Olympics were held June 27–July 2, 1987, in St. Louis, Missouri. Among those participating were some members of the 1936 United States Olympic Team. Competition was held in archery, bowling, cycling, golf, horseshoes, swimming, table tennis, track and field, road race, and volleyball (Figs. 13.1 and 13.2).

In 1986, there were approximately 30 local Senior Games held in the United States; in 1987 about 80 local Games were held. For

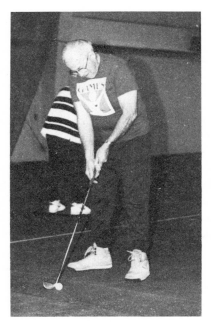

Figure 13.1. Senior Games, golf.

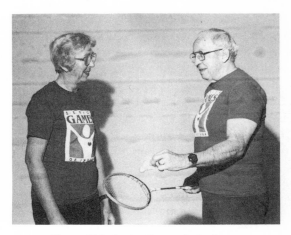

Figure 13.2. Senior Games, badminton.

information about the Games in your area, contact your local Area Agency on Aging of the State Council on Aging. In many states they coordinate the events. Participants usually pay a small fee for registration and sign a waiver. Frequently, commemorative T-shirts are available. Medals are presented to the first, second, and third place finalists in each event. Often there are Health Fairs held at the same time, offering screening for blood pressure, cholesterol, diabetes, and glaucoma as well as vision and hearing tests. Social events are planned in addition to the competitive events and table games. The goal of these Games is to provide an opportunity for those who want to, to compete against others of their own age in a pleasant, safe environment. Check the Resources section for more information.

SPORTING ACTIVITIES

Bowling and golf are two activities that are popular with people of all ages, so if you have enjoyed participating in them over the years, then keep enjoying them now. Bowling can enhance your muscle strength, balance, and coordination and offers the camaraderie of being on a team. Golf, without using a motorized cart, is walking—sort of like a fitness trail—stopping to do an arm, shoulder, back coordination exercise periodically. With golf, you also have the opportunity to enjoy the outdoors. Tennis and badminton, especially doubles, are sports that bring enjoyment to those who have played throughout their adult years.

MASTERS SWIMMING

Now, older swimmers, who used to have to give up competing at an early age, can continue to swim competitively as long as they are willing and able, thanks to the Masters Swimming Program. The Masters group was founded in 1970 by Dr. Ransom Arthur of Los Angeles, a long-time swimmer who believed that adults needed a place to keep swimming. The Masters first national meet, held that year, registered 50 competitors; in 1986, 870 competed. The group represented 46 states and six foreign countries and included several former Olympians. But you needn't be an Olympian to join. In 1990 nearly 27,000 people paid the modest $10.00 fee required to join the program. While many Masters swimmers cite the new friendships they have made as a big reason for staying with the program, most are drawn by the excellent physical benefits swimming offers.

Masters meets are conducted just like any other swim meet, with swimmers seeded by past times and competing in age groups ranging from 25–29 to 85–89. A California woman held 15 world records in 1987 at age 88 and was seriously challenged by another woman of 80. Unlike Olympic or junior competitions, national and world Masters championship meets are open to any swimmer with the time, money, and desire to compete. In 1986, nearly 2400 swimmers attended a national meet at Stanford University, setting an attendance record for any swim meet ever in the United States.

Most larger cities, and some smaller communities as well, have active Masters Swimming Programs. See the Resources section for more information.

VOLKSMARCHE

This popular walking event originated in Germany in 1963 in the small Bavarian town of Bobingen. It began as a running event but was eventually expanded to offer walking, swimming, biking, and snow skiing all under the organization known as the "people's sports" clubs. In 1986, this organization became the Internationaler Volksport Verband (IVV). The IVV has grown to include 13 member countries including the United States. The Walkfest, or Volksmarch (either 10km, 20km, or 42km) is the most popular event. Interest in this organized walking sport has continued to grow so that today, in Germany alone, there may be more than 2000 marches in a single year. American military personnel stationed in Germany have been among the millions that participate there, and when they return to the United States they bring with them their enthusiasm for Volksmarches. By November 1988, there were 58 Volksmarch clubs in the American Volksport Association.

A day at a Volksmarch begins at the registration table where, for a modest fee, you are entitled to a medal commemorating the event when you have completed the hike. You are then ready to follow the signs for the specific distance you have chosen to walk. The marches have a checkpoint midway where your registration card is stamped and where you can also get some refreshment. There are also First Aid personnel available to assist you if necessary. Many times there are bands, music, and dancing to greet you at the Finish Hall where you receive your medal (Fig. 13.3). In Germany, the Volksmarch often ends with a cold drink and a wurst, and the same is often true in this country. Participating in a Volksmarch is something you can do alone or it can be a family event. Either way, it offers you the opportunity to make new friends and have a pleasant exercise outing. Most marches are held in scenic areas so you can enjoy nature and the outdoor surroundings as well.

If this sounds like an activity you might enjoy, see the Resources section for the address of the American Volksport Associa-

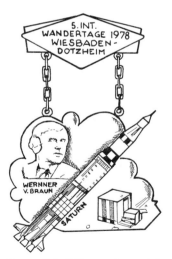

Figure 13.3. Volksmarche medal.

tion. You can also check with your local YMCA to see if they are
sponsoring a local club or know of one in your area.

RACE WALKING

We do not see too many people out race walking, and when
we do we often chuckle at their strange way of "wiggle walking."
Nevertheless, this form of exercise has a long history. It has been
traced back to the 16th century when walking races were held in
England and Europe. It became an international competitive event
at the 1908 Olympic Games. It is gaining in popularity as many
former runners switch to race or speed walking as they grow older.
Speed is not the only component of race walking however; technique is also extremely important. The official definition of race
walking, as stated by the International Amateur Athletic Federa-
tion, is as follows: "Race walking is progression by steps taken so
that unbroken contact with the ground is maintained." In other
words, the front foot must contact the ground before the rear foot
leaves the ground. Also, the knee of the supporting leg must be
straight as it passes under the body. The hip swings forward to
lengthen the stride, and the arms are also moving (Figs. 13.4 and
13.5). The elbows should be bent at a 90° angle and drive in an arc
from the hip, where the side seams of the shorts are, to the mid-
chest. As in normal walking, the right arm is forward when the left
leg is forward.

The benefits are many, since the activity involves the total
body and requires a coordinated effort from the feet, legs, hips,
torso, shoulders, and arms. It requires more involvement of the
abdominal muscles than either running or walking. And, of
course there is the obvious benefit to the cardiovascular system. In
addition, the risk of injuries is much lower than with jogging, for
example. It is recommended, however, that you learn the correct
technique from an experienced race walker. This will help you

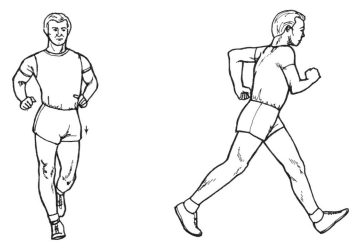

Figure 13.4. Racewalking stride (front).   Figure 13.5. Racewalking stride (side).

keep from developing any bad habits such as holding the shoulders too high or swinging the arms too high, both of which cause tension, fatigue, and strain to the upper body.

Once you have learned the technique and begun, you will find that there is a great sense of camaraderie among race walkers. The rhythmic involvement of the entire body rewards the walker with a pleasant sensation and a feeling of accomplishment. This is an inexpensive sport in which the major considerations are shoes and comfortable clothing. Here again, invest well in a good shoe. You can wear it for years and your feet will thank you for it.

If you think race walking is a sport you would like to try, you can begin by checking the Resources section to find a race walking club in your area.

EXERCISE WITH OTHERS

Even though you have set up your own exercise program, tailored to your personal needs, at some point you may also choose to join a class. When you do, there are several things to consider in making a wise and safe decision. First, go and observe a class. Most will encourage you to participate in one class free of charge, and in this way you can get a feeling for what the program, instructor, and other class members are like.

The following checklist (also listed in Appendix N) to help you make your choice was developed based upon *The Guidelines for*

Table 13.1
Evaluation of an Exercise Program

1. Does the exercise leader have training and experience in working with older adults in exercise? _____ Yes _____ No

2. Is the exercise leader aware of the importance of monitoring each participant's response to exercise?

    Heart Rate _____ Pallor _____ Labored Breathing _____
    Nausea _____ Pain _____

3. Are participants taught to monitor their own heart rates?
    _____ Yes _____No

4. Does the exercise leader have a well-defined emergency plan in the event of cardiac arrest or other accident? _____ Yes _____ No

5. Is there adequate supervision? _____Yes _____No

6. What is the size of the group? _____

7. Is the exercise leader trained in cardiopulmonary resuscitation (CPR) techniques?
    _____Yes _____No

8. Are the participants enjoying themselves and having FUN?
    _____ Yes _____ No

9. Is the exercise facility adequate and safe for older adults to exercise? _____ Yes
    _____ No

Exercise Programs for Older Persons, 1981, by the American Alliance for Health, Physical Education, Recreation and Dance Board of Governors. Use it as you observe any program you may be interested in joining.

A FINAL WORD

These are only a few of the extras that can add to our lives as we grow older. The "golden years" as they are sometimes called, may truly be golden—as full of joy and satisfaction as the younger years. Now, there is a well-earned sense of freedom to at last attend to our own needs and wants. And with better health, longer life, and increasing opportunities for fulfillment, these years can be as rich and rewarding as we choose to make them.

BIBLIOGRAPHY

Suggested Reading

Agne-Traub, C. E., and Traub, G. L., 1987, Volksmarching: A popular leisure activity for the middle-aged, *Journal of Physical Education, Recreation and Dance* **50**(8):59.

Brant, J., 1989, Fifty something: Runners over 50 lead active, fulfilling lives and offer the rest of us know-how and inspiration, *Runners World* **24**(8):58–61.

Gandee, A. N., Knierim, H., Ziegler, A., Campbell, T., Cosky, A., Leslie, D., and Snodgrass, J., 1989, Senior Olympic games: Opportunities for older adults, *Journal of Physical Education, Recreation and Dance* **60**(3):72–76.

Green, R., 1990, Senior tour: Together again, Gary & Arnie & Jack & Lee, *Sports Illustrated* **72**(9):5.

Heldman, G. M., 1989, Senior partners. In making up for lost time, seniors have developed a few tricks all doubles can try, *World Tennis* **36**(11):66, 79.

Higdon, H., 1990, *The Masters Running Guide: Beyond Fitness: How To Get in Shape to Perform for the Best Years of Your Life*, Van Nuys, Calif., National Masters News.

Menard, D., and Stanish, W. D., 1989, The aging athlete, *American Journal of Sports Medicine* **17**(2):187–196.

Moore, K., 1989, The times of their lives: spirits spared and records fell as 4,950 hoary but hale athletes competed at the world veterans' games, *Sports Illustrated* **71**(7):44–47.

Porcari, J., McCarron, A., Kline, G., Freedson, P., Ward, A., Ross, J., and Rippe, J., 1987, Is fast walking an adequate aerobic training stimulus for 30- to 69-year-old men and women? *Physician and Sportsmedicine* **15**(2):119–122, 127–129.

Shea, E. J., 1990, Older americans in sport, *Indiana ANPEAD Journal* **19**(1):38–40.

Teh, J., 1989, Whoa, whippersnapper: An old-timer rises to the defense of senior sports, *Sports Illustrated* **71**(7):90.

Ungerleider, S., Porter, K., Golding, J., and Foster, J., 1989, Mental advantages for masters: A psychological study of 1,014 master athletes finds that some things do improve with age, *Running Times* **July**:18–21.

Wulf, S., 1989, The boys of winter: The senior professional baseball association has plenty of gung ho players, *Sports Illutrated* **71**(21):28–33.

Resources

American Volksport Association, Suite 203, 1001 Pat Booker Rd., Phoenix Square, Universal City, TX 78148; Telephone: (512) 659-1211.

Elderhostel, 75 Federal, 3rd Floor, Boston, MA 02110.

Masters Swim Programs, Dorothy Donnelly, Executive Secretary, U. S. Masters Swimming, 495 Lovely Street, Avon, CT 06001; Telephone: (508) 886-6631.

North American Racewalking Foundation, P.O. Box 50312, Pasadena, CA 91105; West Coast: Elaine Ward, Telephone: (818) 577-2264; East Coast: John MacLachlan, Telephone: (305) 393-6125.

Senior Games Developmental Council, 200 Castlewood Drive, North Palm Beach, FL 33408.

United States Senior Olympics Foundation, 8910 Pine Acre Road, St. Louis, MO 63124.

Appendixes

AAHPERD Council on Aging and Adult Development
Medical/Exercise Assessment for Older Adults[a]

Date _____

Name _____ Age _____ Phone (_____) _____

Street _____ City _____ State _____ Zip _____

Part I—TO BE FILLED OUT BY PARTICIPANT

ACTIVITY HISTORY

1. How would you rate your physical activity level during the last year?
   - ____ Little—Sitting, typing, driving, talking—no exercise planned
   - ____ Mild—Standing, walking, bending, reaching
   - ____ Moderate—Standing, walking, bending, reaching, exercise 1 day per week
   - ____ Active—Light physical work, climbing stairs, exercise 2–3 days per week
   - ____ Very active—Moderate physical work, regular exercise 4 or more days per week
2. What exercise and recreational activities are you presently involved in and how often? _____

HEALTH HISTORY

Weight _____ Height _____ Recent weight loss/gain _____

Please list any recent illnesses: _____

Please list hospitalizations and reasons during last 5 years: _____

Please check the box in front of those conditions which you have experienced.

☐ Anemia
☐ Arthritis/bursitis
☐ Asthma
☐ Blood pressure _____
☐ Bowel/bladder problems
☐ Chest pains
☐ Chest discomfort while exercising
☐ Diabetes
☐ Difficulty with hearing
   _____
☐ Difficulty with vision
   _____
☐ Dizziness or balance problems

☐ Heart conditions _____
☐ Hernia
☐ Indigestion
☐ Joint pain in _____
☐ Leg pain on walking
☐ Lung disease
☐ Shortness of breath
☐ Passing out spells
☐ Osteoporosis _____
☐ Low back condition
☐ Other orthopedic conditions
   [List]
   _____

Smoking:
   Never smoked   Smoke now [how much? _____]   Smoked in past
Alcohol consumption:
   None   Occasional   Often [how much? _____]
List any existing health concerns _____
_____

Please list medication and or dietary supplements you regularly take
_____

PART II—TO BE FILLED OUT BY PHYSICIAN
Date of Last Examination _____

PHYSICAL EXAMINATION—Please check if it applies to the patient.

☐ Resting heart rate _____   ☐ Resting blood pressure
☐ Chest auscultation abnormal   _____
☐ Heart size abnormal   ☐ Thyroid abnormal
☐ Peripheral pulses normal   ☐ Any joints abnormal
☐ Abnormal heart sounds, gal-   ☐ Abnormal mass
  lops   ☐ Other _____
Present prescribed medication[s] _____

CARDIOVASCULAR LABORATORY EXAMINATION
[Within one year of the present date if recommended by physician].
DATE: _____

Resting ECG: Rate _____ Rhythm _____
  Axis _____ Interpretation _____
  Stress test: Max H.R. _____ Max B.P. _____ Total time _____
Max VO$_2$ _____ METS _____ Type of test _____
Recommendation for exercise. Moderate is defined as standing, walking, bending, reaching and light exercise 3 days a week. Please check one.
_____ There is no contraindication to participation in moderate exercise program.
_____ Because of the above analysis, participation in a moderate exercise program may be advisable, but further examination or consultation is necessary, namely: stress test, EKG, other .
_____ Because of the above analysis, my patient may participate only under direct supervision of a physician. [Cardiac rehabilitation program]
_____ Because of the above analysis, participation in a moderate exercise program is inadvisable.

SUMMARY IMPRESSION OF PHYSICIAN

Comments on any history of orthopedic and neuromuscular disorders that may affect participation in an exercise program—especially those checked. _____

_____

Message for the Exercise Program Director: _____

_____

Physician: _____ Signature: _____
            [Please type/print]

Address: _____ Phone: (____) _____

PART III—PATIENT'S RELEASE AND CONSENT

_____ Release: I hereby release the above information to the Exercise Program Director.

_____ Consent: I agree to see my private physician for medical care and agree to have an evaluation by him/her once a year, if necessary.

SIGNATURE: _____ DATE: _____

[a]Form developed by DeeAnn Birkel, Ray Harris, William Martz, and Wayne Osness for American Alliance of Health, Physical Education, Recreation and Dance. Reprinted with permission.

Ball State University Fitness Appraisal Test[a]

NAME _____ AGE _____ DATE _____

	1	2	3
1. Resting pulse (beats per min)			
2. Height (to nearest 1/4 in)			
3. Weight (to nearest lb)			
4. Blood Pressure			
5. Girth Measurements (to nearest 1/2 in)			
Right wrist			
Right upperarm			
Chest			
Waist			
Abdomen			
Hips			
Right thigh			
Right calf			
Right ankle			
6. Percent body fat			
7. Flexibility (inches + or −)			
8. Balance Answer yes or no			
How many sec can I balance on 1 leg?			
Did I show control?			
Did I use my arms to assist me?			
Did I use vision to assist me?			
Did I show good form?			

10. Cardiovascular (Record min and sec and
    beats/min)

    1/2 mile: Pulse   _____

                 Time   _____

    1 mile: Pulse   _____

                 Time   _____

    Rockport category   _____

11. Abdominal curl (record in)   _____

[a]This self appraisal was developed by Dee Ann Birkel and Gwen Robbins of Ball
State University (copyright, 1991.)

Rockport Walking Test[a]

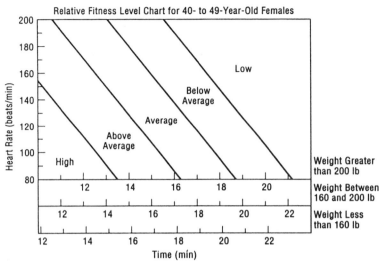

Relative Fitness Level Chart for 40- to 49-Year-Old Females

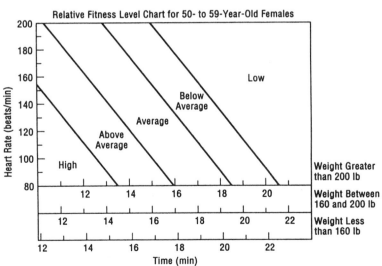

Relative Fitness Level Chart for 50- to 59-Year-Old Females

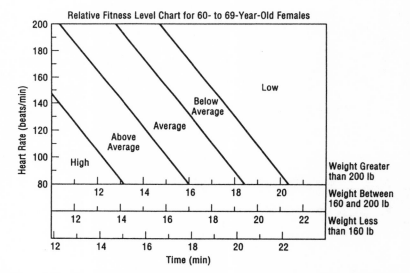

Relative Fitness Level Chart for 60- to 69-Year-Old Females

aFrom the book, *The Rockport Walking Program*, by Dr. James M. Rippe and Ann Ward, Ph.D., with Karla Dougherty, © 1989. Used by permission of the publisher, Prentice Hall Press/A division of Simon & Schuster, New York, NY 10023.

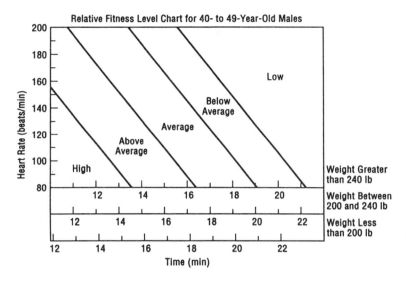

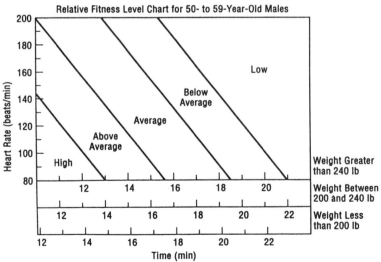

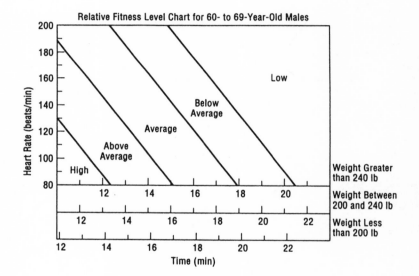

Relative Fitness Level Chart for 60- to 69-Year-Old Males

Personal Goals Record Form

1. Do I want to exercise with other people or do I prefer to exercise by myself? _____

2. What are my personal goals?
   _____ I hope to improve flexibility in my _____, _____, or _____.
   _____ I want to relieve pain in my _____, _____, or _____.
   _____ I need to lose weight. Other. _____

3. I need to tone and strengthen the muscles in my
   _____ abdomen, _____ thighs, _____ arms, _____ feet, _____ back,
   _____ neck and shoulders

4. Do I need to improve my balance? _____

5. Do I need to improve my agility and coordination? _____

6. Do I want a set of exercises I can do in privacy? _____

7. Do I need to learn to handle stress in my life? _____

8. Do I like to: _____ walk, _____ dance, _____ play tennis, _____ cycle,
   _____ swim, _____ do chair exercises, _____ do floor exercises.

9. What else do I want to gain from exercising? _____
   _____

Holmes & Rahe Social Readjustment Rating Scale

The Social Readjustment Rating Scale[a]

Note that both good things, like a marriage or outstanding personal achievement and bad things, like a death or divorce, can cause stress. To figure your risk, add up the total score for all the items which aply to you *for the last year*.

If you score below 150 you are reasonably safe. If your score is between 150 and 300, your odds are about 50/50 for experiencing a significant health change within the next two years. Finally, if you scored above 300 points, great caution is suggested. According to some interpretations, the chances of your having a serious illness or accident in the next two years are roughly 80 percent. Some stress intervention and a "pulling back" from a life of rapid change is strongly suggested.

Life event	Mean value
1. Death of spouse	100
2. Divorce	73
3. Marital separation	65
4. Jail term	63
5. Death of close family member	63
6. Personal injury or illness	53
7. Marriage	50
8. Fired at work	47
9. Marital reconciliation	45
10. Retirement	45
11. Change in health of family member	44
12. Pregnancy	40
13. Sex difficulties	39
14. Gain of new family member	39
15. Business readjustment	39
16. Change in financial state	38

Life event	Mean value
17. Death of close friend	37
18. Change to different line of work	36
19. Change in number of arguments with spouse	35
20. Mortgage over $10,000	31
21. Foreclosure of mortgage or loan	30
22. Change in responsibilities at work	29
23. Son or daughter leaving home	29
24. Trouble with in-laws	29
25. Outstanding personal achievement	28
26. Wife begins or stops work	26
27. Beginning or ending school	26
28. Change in living conditions	25
29. Revision of personal habits	24
30. Trouble with boss	23
31. Change in work hours or conditions	20
32. Change in residence	20
33. Change in schools	20
34. Change in recreation	19
35. Change in church activities	19
36. Change in social activities	18
37. Mortgage or loan less than $10,000	17
38. Change in sleeping habits	16
39. Change in number of family get-togethers	15
40. Change in eating habits	15
41. Vacation	13
42. Christmas	12
43. Minor violations of the law	11

[a]See Holmes, T. H. and Rahe, R. H., 1967, The Social Readjustment Rating Scale, *Journal of Psychosomatic Research* **11:**213–218 for complete wording of the items.

Checklist for Shoe Purchase

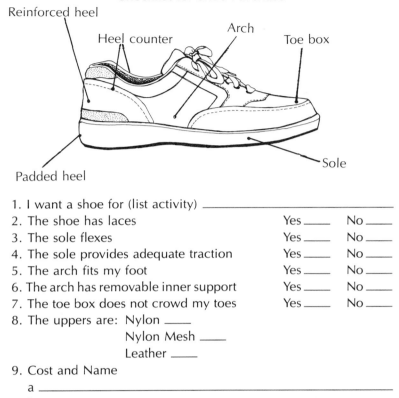

Reinforced heel

Heel counter

Arch

Toe box

Padded heel

Sole

1. I want a shoe for (list activity) _____
2. The shoe has laces   Yes _____   No _____
3. The sole flexes   Yes _____   No _____
4. The sole provides adequate traction   Yes _____   No _____
5. The arch fits my foot   Yes _____   No _____
6. The arch has removable inner support   Yes _____   No _____
7. The toe box does not crowd my toes   Yes _____   No _____
8. The uppers are: Nylon _____
                    Nylon Mesh _____
                    Leather _____
9. Cost and Name
    a _____
    b _____
    c _____

Exercise Program Worksheet

1. Physician's comments and recommendations _____
   _____
   _____
2. I need to be concerned about _____
   _____
3. I enjoy doing _____
4. My personal goals are _____
5. The proper attire is _____
6. I need to _____ lose or _____ gain _____ pounds.
7. I will include a stress-reduction activity of _____
8. The medications I take may affect me during exercise.
   Yes _____ No _____. If yes, how will it affect me? _____
   _____
9. I need to improve flexibility in my (list body areas) _____,
   _____ , _____ , _____ , _____
10. I need to improve muscle strength and endurance in my (list
    body areas) _____ , _____ ,
    _____ , _____ , _____
11. I need to improve my balance. Yes _____ No _____
12. I plan to participate in _____ to improve my cardio-
    respiratory endurance.
13. My body composition needs improvement in the following
    ways _____
    _____
14. To calculate the intensity level of my exercise workout:
    I. Resting pulse _____ + 20 beats = _____ .
    II. Estimate of maximal heart rate:

	220	220
	−Age	−55
Predicted maximal heart rate		165
Percent intensity	× %	(50%) ×
		0.5
Training or target heart rate		82.5

8. Kneeling on mat or padded floor do:
   a. Cat, #21, beg.: 4, chal.: 8, (p. 116)
9. Lying on back on mat or padded floor do:
   a. Knees to Chest, #17, beg.: 5, chal.: 10, (p. 112)

Basic Cool-down Program

1. Walk at a slower pace, or if riding on an exercise bike, ride at a slower pace.

Standing, do:

2. Single Arm Swings, #5; beg.:5, chal.:10; (p. 103)
3. Wall Walk and Slide, #7; beg.:2–4, chal.:6; (p. 104)
4. Shoulder Shrugs, #9; beg.:2–4, chal.:6; (p. 106)
5. Chest Stretch in Doorway, #13; beg.:3 each side, chal.:6; (p. 110)
6. Lower Leg Stretch at Wall, #30; beg.:3 each leg, chal.:6 each leg; (p. 123)

Lying on padded floor or mat do:

7. Knees to Chest, #17a,b; beg.:5, chal.:8; (p. 112)
8. Crocodile Twist, #18; beg.:4, chal.:8; (p. 114)
9. Knee-overs, #19; beg.:4 to each side, chal.:8 to each side; (p. 114)
10. Pose of Child, #22; both beg. and chal. stay as long as comfortable; (p. 116)

Record of Progressive Conditioning Program

Date	Begin pulse[a]	Warm up	Pulse[a]	Mode[b]	Dis-tance/ intensity	Time	Exer-cise pulse[a]	Cool down

[a]Count pulse for 6 sec, add a zero, and record.
[b]Walking: W; Stationary bike: SB; Swimming: SW; Walking/jogging: WJ; Dancing: D; Jogging: J; Yoga: Y; Tai Ji: TJ; Aquatic: AQ.

Resistance Training Record Form

Exercise/ station no.	sets	Date								
1. Quadriceps		wgt reps								
2. Hamstrings		wgt reps								
3. Leg crossovers		wgt reps								
4. Lat or deltoid		wgt reps								
5. Bench press		wgt reps								
6. Biceps		wgt reps								
7. Triceps		wgt reps								

Record of Progressive Cycling Program

Workout day and activity	Begin pulse[a]	Warm up stretch-ing	Half-way pulse[a]	Dis-tance	Resis-tance on exer-cycle	Time	End pulse[a]	Cool down

[a]Count pulse for 6 sec, add a zero, and record.

Swimming Record Form

Date	Laps	Continuous swimming Distance	Time	Pulse rate Halfway	End of cont. swim	Total work-out time

Evaluation of an Exercise Program

1. Does the exercise leader have training and experience in working with older adults in exercise? ____ Yes ____ No
2. Is the exercise leader aware of the importance of monitoring each participant's response to exercise?
   Heart rate ____
   Pallor ____
   Labored breathing ____
   Nausea ____
   Pain ____
3. Are participants taught to monitor their own heart rates?
   ____ Yes ____ No
4. Does the exercise leader have a well-defined emergency plan in the event of cardiac arrest or other accident? ____ Yes ____ No
5. Is there adequate supervision? ____ Yes ____ No
6. What is the size of the group? _____
7. Is the exercise leader trained in cardiopulmonary resuscitation (CPR) techniques? ____ Yes ____ No
8. Are the participants enjoying themselves and having fun?
   ____ Yes ____ No
9. Is the exercise facility adequate and safe for older adults to exercise? ____ Yes ____ No

Index

Back, exercises for
back push-up, 115
cat, 116
crocodile twist, 114
knee-overs, 114–115
knees to chest, 112–113
pelvic tilt, 112, 121
pose of the child, 116–117
Balance, 28
Basic cool down, 134, 293
Basic 40 exercises, 100–132
Basic four food groups, 52–54
Basic warm up, 133, 291–292
Benson, Herbert, 161
Bent-knee sit-ups, 90
Birdie dance, 224–225
Blood pressure, 24–25
Body–brain mechanics, 151–153
Body composition, 17
Body fat, percentage of, 26
Bowling, 263
Breathing
proper pattern, 81
relaxation and, 159–161
vital capacity and, 18
BSU Self-Appraisal, 23–31, 93
Buttocks, exercises for
buttock firmer, 121
kneeling single leg lifts, 122
pelvic tilt, 112–121

Calipers, 26
Cardiorespiratory efficiency, 18–19
Cardiovascular disease, 37, 41–42
Cataracts, 40, 43–44
Cha-Cha, 219
Chair dancing, 217
Checklists
exercise class, 268
safety, 86
shoe purchase, 68
stationary bike, 208
Chest, exercises for
chest expansion, 143–144

Chest, exercises for (cont.)
chest stretch in doorway, 109
forearm press isometrically, 111
wall push-up, 110
Clothing, 64–65
Competitive activities
Masters Swimming, 263–264
Senior Olympics, 260–262
Cool down
for aquatic exercise
beginner level, 244–247
challenge level, 251–252
basic, 134, 293
definition of, 20
for fitness swimming, 255–256
guidelines for, 77
Cotton-Eyed Joe, 222
Cycling
equipment for, 207–208
guidelines for, 205–207
precautions, 207
program for, 209
record-keeping for, 210
road, 209
stationary, 205–209
warm up and cool down for, 206–207

Dancer's plié, 89, 126, 231
Dancing
attire for, 216–217
ballet, 228–233
benefits of, 214–215
chair (jarming), 217
country western, 221–224
folk, 219–221
guidelines for, 215–216
line, 224–227
low-impact aerobic, 228
social (ballroom), 217–219
Deep knee bends, 89
deVries, Herbert, 4
Diabetes, 36–37, 41
Diastolic pressure, 24–25

About the Authors

Dee Ann Green Birkel, M.A., is an Assistant Professor at the School of Physical Education, Ball State University, Muncie, Indiana. She is also Director of the BSU Retirees Exercise Program, in which older adults return to campus to exercise with college students who are specializing in Physical Activity for the Older Adult. Ms. Birkel has long been involved in the national organization of the American Alliance of Health, Physical Education, Recreation, and Dance, serving on its committees for the Council

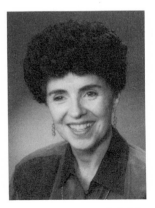
Dee Ann Green Birkel, M.A.

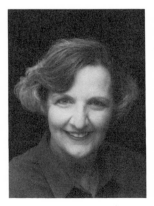
Susan Birkel Freitag, M.S.

on Aging and Adult Development. She has taught yoga and dance to Elderhostelers and given many presentations in the areas of fitness, hatha yoga, and older adult exercise in the United States and abroad. Ms. Birkel is also the author of *Hatha Yoga: Developing the Body, Mind, and Inner Self* (Eddie Bowers Publishing, 1991).

Susan Birkel Freitag, M.S., has spent more than 25 years working as a medical/scientific writer and editor at the Texas Medical Center in Houston, one of the nation's largest medical centers. She earned her master's degree in biomedical sciences from the University of Texas Health Science Center at Houston and underwent subsequent extensive training in biomedical communications, health sciences, and medical terminology. A member of and panelist for the American Medical Writers Association, Ms. Freitag currently acts as a freelance medical editor and writer for clients connected with major medical centers and in private practice.